NUTRITIONAL SURVEILLANCE

JOHN B. MASON
Director,
Cornell Nutritional
Surveillance Program,
Ithaca, NY, USA

JEAN-PIERRE HABICHT
Professor
of Nutritional Epidemiology,
Cornell University,
Ithaca, NY, USA

H. TABATABAI
Research Associate,
Cornell Nutritional
Surveillance Program,
Ithaca, NY, USA

V. VALVERDE
Coordinator,
Food and Nutrition Planning,
Institute of Nutrition
of Central America and Panama,
Guatemala

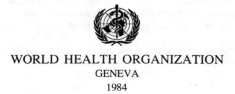
WORLD HEALTH ORGANIZATION
GENEVA
1984

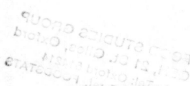

ISBN 92 4 156078 9

© World Health Organization 1984

PRINTED IN BELGIUM

83/5732 – Vanmelle – 6000

CONTENTS

ACKNOWLEDGEMENTS

This book is based on a background document prepared for an International Workshop on Nutritional Surveillance, held in July 1981 in Cali, Colombia. The workshop was sponsored and supported financially by the United Nations Administrative Committee on Coordination – Subcommittee on Nutrition; and was also supported by the Foundation for Higher Education (FES) of Colombia, the Agency for Technical Cooperation (GTZ) of the Federal Republic of Germany, the Kellogg Foundation, the Pan American Health Organization, the United States Agency for International Development, the University of Valle, and the World Health Organization.

The first version was prepared in 1981 by the Cornell Nutritional Surveillance Program – Director, John B. Mason; Assistant-Director, Hamid Tabatabai – with the guidance of Professor J.-P. Habicht and Professor M.C. Latham. Other programme staff involved in the preparation of the first manuscript were Terry Elliott, Maarten Immink, Robert Jackson, Cay Loria, Janice Mitchell, and June Wolgemuth. A revised version was used at a workshop convened jointly by Cornell University and UNICEF, on Social and Nutritional Surveillance in Eastern and Southern Africa, in May 1982, in Nairobi, Kenya.

The authors wish to acknowledge the substantial contribution to Chapter 1 by David O. Dapice, Associate Professor of Economics, Tufts University. We also greatly appreciate the helpful comments of many colleagues who have reviewed the draft in its many stages, including: D.J. Casley, D.O. Dapice, A. Horwitz, J. Kreysler, J. McKigney, P. Payne, E. Thorbecke, and K. Williams.

The authors especially wish to thank Janice Mitchell, for revising the final text, and Sondra Palmer for transferring it into the word processor.

We owe particular thanks to Dr John McKigney, Office of Nutrition, USAID, for his crucial support to nutritional surveillance and to the programme at Cornell; and to Dr M.C. Nesheim, Director of the Division of Nutritional Sciences, for enabling the work to be carried out at Cornell.

Finally, and most important, we wish gratefully to acknowledge the unstinting help of many colleagues in many countries and international agencies, who have frankly discussed their experiences and views with us, and agreed to our drawing on this information. Without their long-term efforts in nutrition, development, and health, there would be no such thing as nutritional surveillance, and no experience to build upon.

The Cornell Nutritional Surveillance Program is supported by a Cooperative Agreement with the Office of Nutrition, USAID (No. AID DSAN CA-0240) between the Office of Nutrition, Bureau of Science and Technology, USAID, and the Division of Nutritional Sciences, New York State Colleges of Human Ecology and Agriculture and Life Sciences, Cornell University, Ithaca, New York.

Preface

In most developing countries, the balance between an adequate level of nutrition and severe malnutrition is finely poised. Relatively minor changes in the economic situation or in environmental factors can upset this balance and precipitate widespread protein-energy malnutrition. There is therefore a need for programmes that will monitor the nutritional status of the population, ensure timely warning of impending shortages in food consumption, and instigate both long-term and short-term measures to prevent such crises or, at least, to alleviate them. These are the purposes of nutritional surveillance.

The first chapter of this book examines the role of nutritional surveillance. It discusses a number of planning considerations and the relation of health, nutrition and basic needs to different development strategies. It also outlines the types of action that can be taken to improve nutrition and the various data requirements. A procedure for deciding the precise purpose of nutritional surveillance and hence the way in which the system might operate is described in Chapter 2. This deals with initial assessment and should provide guidance on the priorities that will subsequently require attention. In the next two chapters, the principles that apply to all the purposes of nutritional surveillance are set out in detail. For example, the users need to be identified, the organizational structures set up, outputs decided upon, and data sources selected. Chapter 5 covers considerations specific to evaluation and develops theories to guide systems aimed at this objective. Timely warning and intervention programmes, which are described in Chapter 6, differ in a number of respects from the other two types of surveillance, particularly in regard to organization and data requirements.

The book is organized primarily to cater for the needs of practitioners of nutritional surveillance, i.e., those directly involved in planning and evaluating measures to improve nutrition. However, it is hoped that others concerned in more general ways with nutrition will also find some of the information useful. They may wish to skip some sections, such as those on organizational details, but may find it useful to consider both the theory of the different uses of the information collected and the examples given of data that have been used for different purposes.

CHAPTER 1

The role of nutritional surveillance in tackling nutrition and health problems

Summary

Activities that have come to be known as nutritional surveillance constitute one of several ways of gaining the knowledge required to ensure adequate nutrition. Nutritional surveillance means keeping watch over nutrition in order to make decisions that will lead to improvement in nutrition in populations. The concept stems from disease surveillance, with which it has several principles in common, but it is related to a wider range of possible actions in several sectors of government. The focus in this book is on actions to alleviate protein-energy malnutrition in developing countries.

Recently, the purposes of nutritional surveillance have been defined as: health and development planning, usually at national level; programme management and evaluation; and timely warning and intervention to prevent short-term food consumption crises. These purposes are not mutually exclusive, but impose different requirements on the design of nutritional surveillance systems. They provide the basic structure of this book.

The need for nutritional surveillance stems from the recognition that the major cause of malnutrition in the world is poverty. Poverty causes malnutrition through inadequate food availability in households (and perhaps inappropriate distribution within the household) and through insanitary living conditions and inadequate access to health services. These interrelations can be regarded as flows of resources determining nutritional status as an endpoint. This concept helps to define points of intervention and data needs.

Improvement in nutrition is one of the objectives of basic needs planning, of health for all, and of food and nutrition planning. The measurements used in nutritional surveillance include many of those defined as health status indicators, particularly with respect to the nutritional status of children and mortality data. The same measurements are useful for assessing the effects of development programmes.

A feasible strategy for tackling health and nutrition problems involves: enhancing the positive effects on nutrition of development policies and programmes that are already occurring or being planned for primarily economic and political reasons; rationalizing and effectively carrying out specific targeted programmes mainly in the conventional health and nutrition fields; and preventing short-term critical reductions in food consumption. Support for this strategy is the main *raison d'être* of nutritional surveillance. Success depends on numerous considerations, many of which are political, but knowledge of nutritional problems, their causes and how they are changing, can help in many relevant decisions.

Decisions are required in the context of both national policies and particular programmes. Decisions on national policies concern resource allocation by area and sector, legislative measures (e.g., prices), and programmes. Nutritional surveillance provides for better-informed decisions within these areas. Development programmes require choices on targeting by area and socioeconomic group, and on the possible effects of different activities on nutrition. Health and nutrition programmes need similar decisions: on targeting by area, and on relevance of activities to causes of malnutrition. Timely warning and intervention programmes to tackle acute food shortages need data to trigger appropriate interventions.

What is Nutritional Surveillance?

Adequate nutrition is a basic human need and a prerequisite for health. Promotion of proper nutrition is one of the eight essential elements of primary health care (*1*, pp. 24 and 34). Public policy decisions on nutrition – in health and other sectors – require knowledge about the extent to which people consume sufficient food of adequate quality, the effects of infectious diseases, how these relate to human health and wellbeing, and the determinants of these factors (*2*, pp. 28-32). Such knowledge is derived in many ways and the ways that are encompassed by the term ''nutritional surveillance'' represent only some of these. This section sketches out the boundaries of what nutritional surveillance has come to mean.

Nutritional surveillance could be concerned with everything that affects nutrition, from food production, distribution and intake to health status itself. Indeed, the World Food Conference in 1974 proposed that ''global'' nutritional surveillance should be concerned with ''all factors which influence food consumption patterns and nutritional status'' (*3*, p. 9 – Resolution V.13). Such a mandate is in practice self-defeating because it gives no guidance on priorities and a virtually unlimited amount of data would be needed to fulfil it. The priority should be to focus only on data necessary for making important decisions. Data that are not essential for such decisions are not considered to be within the context of nutritional surveillance, however useful they may be for other purposes. Our focus is therefore restricted to the data needed to make decisions on public policies and programmes to ensure adequate nutrition in populations.

Nutritional surveillance is relevant to both under- and overnutrition, and to both industrialized and low-income countries. The focus here is on undernutrition in low-income countries, in line with the goal of ''health for all by the year 2000'', because this is by far the most extensive nutrition problem in the world today. This is not to deny that further expansion of knowledge from nutritional surveillance to other nutritional problems is both desirable and necessary.

Some important activities do not fall within the purview of nutritional surveillance, even though they may be needed for the design of programmes in general terms. For example, fundamental knowledge of cause–effect relationships is the concern of scientific research. A distinguishing characteristic of scientific research is that it is most productive when it is tailored to the scientific question at hand, and this involves not just the measurement process itself, but also the selection of persons to be measured. There is no general data collection procedure that can efficiently collect data to demonstrate cause–effect relationships. Therefore, experimental field studies are not within the scope of this book, although they may be essential for designing improvements in population nutrition, for data collection for nutritional surveillance, for interpreting data, and for other purposes.

Decisions relating to patient diagnosis and management are important for the individual, but they fall outside the scope of nutritional surveillance because they are not directed specifically to decisions about populations. On the other hand, data used for individual patient identification and treatment, such as data collected in screening programmes, in outpatient clinics, or from hospital admission records can sometimes be included in a nutritional surveillance system. Decisions about instituting and managing a screening programme may also draw on nutritional information.

What is nutritional surveillance then? Based on the definition of surveillance given by a Joint FAO/UNICEF/WHO Expert Committee (4, p. 9), we can say that "nutritional surveillance means to watch over nutrition, in order to make decisions which will lead to improvements in nutrition in populations." Nutritional surveillance methods provide regular information about nutrition in populations; they draw data from the most suitable sources that are already available, including surveys and administrative data. The undertaking of *ad hoc* investigations can also be included in nutritional surveillance activities.

Some of the characteristics of surveillance in a public health context are also relevant to nutritional surveillance. In public health work, data may be obtained actively by deliberate collection, and passively by using whatever relevant sources are available. Furthermore, the information is gathered only to the extent necessary to maintain health or control disease. One particular difference between the two lies in the characteristics of the resulting action. For malnutrition, which pervades much of the population in low-income countries, the causality is complex and closely related to poverty (2, p. 20; 5). The range of possible actions to prevent and alleviate malnutrition is extensive, and although often not well-defined, extends beyond the health sector. Nutritional surveillance is therefore relevant to a number of different sectors of government. Health itself is dependent on social and economic development (1, p. 23). Development of primary health care requires intersectoral efforts (1, p. 40), and the managerial and planning process requires adequate and relevant information support.[1] Nutritional surveillance is regarded as an important means of providing such information, and it is a "responsibility of the health sector to participate and cooperate in the establishment and operation of a food and nutrition surveillance system" (2, pp. 9, 27, 31).

The term "nutritional surveillance" first found wide currency following the World Food Conference in 1974. Disease surveillance had become a well-accepted concept (6, 7), and the concept was transferred to nutrition; in the United States of America nutritional surveillance had already begun (8). The idea had also been proposed in the context of drought relief (9). The response of UNICEF, FAO, and WHO to the World Food Conference resolution on nutritional surveillance was, in the first instance, to call a Joint Expert Commit-

---

[1] *Report of a Meeting of Investigators on Methodology of Nutritional Surveillance*, Geneva, World Health Organization, 1978 (unpublished document), p. 57.

tee meeting in 1975; the report of this meeting was entitled *Methodology of nutritional surveillance (4)*. This laid out procedures – at that stage hypothetical and rather ambitious – for establishing nutritional surveillance systems to meet a wide range of objectives. These included describing the character and magnitude of nutrition problems and changes in these; analysis of causes and associated factors to permit a selection of preventive measures, which may or may not be nutritional; support for government decisions on priorities and resource allocations; predictions on probable evolution of nutritional problems, to assist formulation of policy; and monitoring and evaluation of programmes (*4*, p. 9). WHO was nominated to take the lead among the international agencies concerned, and these, with certain bilateral agencies, provided some assistance to several developing countries.

Nutritional surveillance programmes began to be established in developing countries from about 1976 onward. The experience of these programmes provides the main source of information for the present book. The information from these programmes was first brought together in 1980 by the United Nations (Working Group on Nutritional Surveillance of the ACC-SCN) and a group under the National Academy of Sciences, USA (Task Force on Nutritional Surveillance). [1] Previous to that, a number of consultative meetings had been convened by WHO and by regional bodies [2-4] (see also ref. *30*).

Both the ACC-SCN and National Academy of Sciences groups produced definitions of various types of surveillance. These were deliberately similar, and were used to focus attention on the need to distinguish different approaches. A summary of the definitions is given in Table 1.1. The information from these reviews was used to produce a first draft of the present book, entitled *Nutritional surveillance – review of progress,* which was used for an international workshop on nutritional surveillance held in Cali, Colombia, under the auspices of the ACC-SCN in July 1981. [5] The present version incorporates further information from the Cali meeting and results of additional research.

The Joint Expert Committee report *Methodology of nutritional surveillance (4)* thus provided a starting-point in nutritional surveillance. The present book differs from it in several respects. First, it is based primarily on experience and

[1] *Report of the third meeting of the ACC/SCN Working Group on Nutritional Surveillance, Geneva, 24-26 June 1980* (mimeographed document); *Draft report of Task Force Meetings, Food and Nutrition Board, National Academy of Sciences,* Washington, DC, National Academy of Sciences, 1980 (mimeographed document).

[2] Documentation report: *Strategy for nutrition surveillance for ASEAN, 28-30 July 1976, Makati, Philippines.* Manila, National Nutrition Council, 1976.

[3] *Report of the second meeting of the ACC/SCN Working Group on Nutritional Surveillance, Rome, December 1979* (mimeographed document).

[4] *Report of a Meeting of Investigators on Methodology of Nutrition Surveillance,* Geneva, World Health Organization, 1978 (unpublished document); *Workshop on Systems for Monitoring and Predicting Community Nutritional Status, 29 March-5 April 1978, Manila, Philippines,* Manila, WHO Regional Office for the Western Pacific, 1978 (unpublished document ICP/NUT/002)

[5] *Report of the International Workshop on Nutritional Surveillance held in Cali, Colombia, 14-17 July, 1981,* Rome, ACC-SCN, 1982 (document SCN 82/10).

only where this is missing are suggestions made on less-tried grounds. Secondly, and as a result, it is intended to provide more "nuts and bolts" details. Thirdly, it takes account of several important policy decisions that have been formulated since 1975, particularly the policy on primary health care (*1*); the integrating concept of basic needs (*10*); the recognition that economic planning and development policies must take nutritional considerations into account (*2, 5*); and the increasing trend to use nutritional indicators to measure quality of life, specifically as a means of evaluating both development programmes (e.g., ref. *11*, p. 45) and health programmes (*12*, p. 21). Many of the indicators and their sources commonly used in nutritional surveillance are the same as the socioeconomic and health status indicators recommended for monitoring progress in health (*13*, pp. 22-54). Nutritional status of children is now regarded as a central indicator for monitoring progress towards health for all at programme (*12*, p. 21), national (*14*, p. 31), and global levels (*15*, p. 76).

Finally, the pre-eminent importance of actually using information for decision-making is intended to guide all the principles and practices discussed. This book therefore aims to provide enough information to allow those concerned with nutrition – both as an objective of broad policies and programmes, and specifically in relation to health and nutrition interventions – to decide: (*a*) in general terms, on how to proceed in this field; and (*b*) in specific terms, what steps need to be taken in particular situations.

In this book, nutritional surveillance activities are classified by purpose. The different purposes are defined in Table 1.1 and the relationships between them are as follows. The most common use is for health and development planning ((*a*) in Table 1.1) and this may be at national or programme level; if at programme level, it is relevant both to development programmes and to public health and nutrition programmes ((*b*) in Table 1.1). At programme level more localized nutritional surveillance systems are relevant, primarily to support the management of these programmes; use of nutritional surveillance information for evaluation and management is as yet usually not feasible at the national level. Nutritional surveillance for programme management and evaluation is thus a subset of the more general type of nutritional surveillance used for planning. It can be either one part of a national surveillance programme or a localized self-contained activity; in either case it has some of the same aspects as the more general systems of planning, but it requires some modification with respect to organization, linkage to decision-making, and data requirements. One purpose of nutritional surveillance has received particular attention – that related to early warning and intervention ((*c*) in Table 1.1); conceptually, it is similar to other surveillance programmes, but it has certain distinguishing features and needs to be considered separately. As discussed later, we now refer to "timely" rather than "early" warning.

Most of the present experience and many of the principles of nutritional surveillance can be seen from the "general" type of system, with planning as its main purpose. Hence, this book describes systems thoroughly in relation to

Table 1.1. Definitions of terms used in nutritional surveillance [a]

Term	Definition	Comments
(a) Long-term nutrition monitoring	An on-going description of nutrition conditions in the population (with particular attention to subgroups defined in socioeconomic terms as functional groups) – sometimes referred to – for purposes of planning (often at national level), analysing the effects of policies and programmes on nutrition problems, and predicting future trends.	The response to information is relatively slow and is usually either through large-scale national programmes specifically aimed at improving nutrition and health or through inserting nutrition concerns into more general development policies, or both.
(b) Evaluation of programme impact	The monitoring of changes in nutrition indicators consequent on the implementation of programmes that have as objectives an impact on nutrition or, more generally, on satisfaction of basic needs.	The main purpose of this monitoring should be to allow control and improvement of programmes during implementation, through possible improvement in targeting, and by assessing whether intensification or modification of activities is required to obtain the desired impact. Responses to this type of surveillance activity are more immediate than for long-term monitoring in that they involve control of specific programmes.
(c) Timely warning and intervention systems	Surveillance systems aimed at the prevention or alleviation of epidemic inadequacies in food consumption.	Nutrition surveillance of this type is distinguished from long-term monitoring in that it is not directed towards chronic inadequacies in food consumption and malnutrition, but focuses entirely on prevention or alleviation of short-term worsening of nutritional status in vulnerable populations. The basic requirement of such a system is that there exists a mechanism to respond to results predicting potential problems, so that interventions can be mobilized *before* there is a decrease in food consumption. Such systems deal with immediate problems through rapidly mobilizable, short-term interventions.

[a] Adapted from: *Nutritional surveillance: a synopsis (49)*.

existing knowledge and planning, and then picks out additional issues related to the two subtypes: evaluation and management, and timely warning and intervention programmes.

The Role of Nutritional Surveillance

Causes of malnutrition

People are malnourished because they have consumed insufficient food and/or because they are sick. Their food consumption depends on the food available to the household and its distribution within the household. Inadequate food availability may be due to lack of income for purchasing food, often coupled with insufficient production of food. Conditions within poor households may prevent the best nutritional use of the available food and can certainly cause high rates of infection. While inadequate household food availability has in the past been attributed primarily to insufficient national food production and problems of marketing and storage, these factors are now considered to be generally less significant than poverty, which is the major cause of malnutrition. Availability of food to the family is a necessary but not always a sufficient condition for preventing malnutrition because cultural factors may affect use of the available food (2, p. 33).

The factors causing malnutrition are usefully classified as, first, "food" and "non-food" (see ref. 2, p. 33) and second, those affecting the household as a whole, compared with those operating within the household. These are shown in Fig. 1.1 (which is discussed in more detail later): "food" factors largely determine dietary intake, and the "non-food" factors whether the individual is free from infection. These two pathways have a common antecedent in *poverty* (e.g., as represented by income in Fig. 1.1).

Possible measures to reduce malnutrition may thus often be the same as those aimed at reducing poverty itself – through growth in real income and increasing equality of income distribution. It is sometimes argued that it may be more feasible politically to direct increases in income preferentially to the poor than to take measures to redistribute income and assets more directly; poverty-oriented development programmes have just this objective.

Although increased income is generally associated with increased food intake, there are some situations in which the expected relationship changes. When income sources change, as when farmers shift from food to cash crops, nutrition may suffer, for example, if purchased food does not adequately replace that previously obtained from the farm. On the other hand, there may be opportunities for greater impact on the nutrition of households than the net-income effects alone would suggest: through food subsidies or food distribution programmes, for example. Programmes may also be aimed at influencing the allocation of food within the household to the benefit of those – often the children – with the lowest share in relation to their requirements. Additional measures may therefore be needed to ensure that an increase in real income leads to greater household food availability, and sometimes to ensure that this food availability leads to better individual nutrition.

Poverty is usually associated with insanitary living conditions and inadequate health care. Here again, alleviation of poverty is necessary to attack the root causes of poor health and nutrition. Health services and environmental sanitation are effective in reducing malnutrition to the extent that they deal with diseases involved in the causation of malnutrition; and that they reach those populations and individuals in need. To a considerable extent, this means reaching vulnerable groups (mothers, infants, preschool children) among the poor. Providing adequate population coverage is an essential concern of primary health care.

These interrelations can be expressed as a flow of resources determining nutritional status, and this concept has been helpful in developing methods of nutritional surveillance. A typical expression of the concept is shown in Fig. 1.1. The model indicates causative factors affecting nutritional status, and shows points at which interventions may be directed. For our purposes it also lays out the different types of data that are potentially useful for nutritional surveillance. These are discussed in detail in Chapter 4.

Fig. 1.1. Relation of resource and flow variables to nutritional outcome [a]

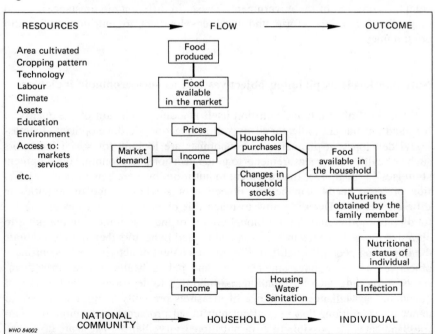

[a] Adapted from ref. 4

One drawback to a presentation such as that in Fig. 1.1 is that it represents a flow in two dimensions and does not emphasize distributional aspects: the flow actually converges from national or area level, then through households to the individual. Maldistribution of available resources between areas, households, and individuals is a central cause of malnutrition (see, for example, ref. *16*). Another feature of this conceptual framework is that it emphasizes technical questions of resource allocation and flow without stressing the social and political environment within which these take place. Conclusions on causality and hence feasible points of intervention depend on the perspective taken. One argument has it that, for example, inequitable distibution of resources (land, capital, education, etc.) is in many circumstances so decisive a cause of poverty and malnutrition that piecemeal measures designed to cope with a particular problem are unlikely to be effective unless major structural change brings about a more receptive environment; worse, direct interventions may even be counter-productive since in the long run they may impede the major changes required. At the other end of the spectrum, possibilities may exist for intervening to tackle the immediate causes of malnutrition. By a more efficient approach to implementing direct, corrective measures, it is argued that inroads on the problem of malnutri-tion can be made even without radical changes. Thus, while nutritional consid-erations might on occasion contribute to decisions on structural changes, the main focus in this book is on policies and programmes that are the current or potential concerns of the government. These, in different circumstances, could range from agrarian reform and rural development to nutrition and health programmes.

Nutrition levels as planning objectives and as socioeconomic indicators

"The level of health and nutrition itself is a direct indicator of the quality of life, and an indirect indicator of overall socioeconomic development. Increas-ingly, development planners and economists are looking for social indicators such as health status measurements to guide decisions on economic development strategies" (*13*, p. 13). Improvement in nutrition, or more generally in satisfac-tion of basic needs, can be one objective of a whole range of activities in different sectors. Deciding how to reach this objective involves assessing the food consumption and the nutritional effects of these activities, and seeking to optimize them. Changes in nutrition and related indicators then help to evaluate the impact on people's quality of life, in the context of activities whose primary objectives are economic, and nutrition and public health programmes them-selves; providing such information and linking it to decisions is the function of nutritional surveillance. The range of measures presently being undertaken, or under consideration, that may affect nutritional problems in developing coun-tries, indicates the possible roles of nutritional surveillance. These are discussed later in this chapter (see also Table 1.3).

Food and nutrition planning has provided one focus for efforts to improve nutrition through wide-ranging actions. At the time of the World Food Conference in 1974, procedures were proposed that were to encompass and guide large areas of government policy-making; these early suggestions may have been overstated since they have not been adopted or implemented. The principles are still accepted, and the main problem has been fitting these in with other government priorities. Thus, in 1974, FAO and WHO (*17*, p. 18) proposed a strategy with three elements: first, broadly-based rural development that would improve production and income distribution; secondly, improvement in the combination of foods produced and their processing and distribution; and thirdly, targeted intervention programmes. Further discussion of the principles and practice is available in, for example, articles by Taylor (*18*), Field (*20*), and Lynch (*21*).

Nutrition objectives have more recently been incorporated in the concepts of "basic needs" and "health for all". Basic needs include two elements: "First, they include certain minimum requirements of a family for private consumption: adequate food, shelter and clothing are obviously included, as would be certain household equipment and furniture. Second, they include essential services provided by and for the community at large, such as safe drinking-water, sanitation, public transport, and health and educational facilities" (*22*, p. 32).

The goal of health for all, to be achieved through primary health care, stresses the need for adequate coverage of services and access to resources to provide for the health needs of all. Health is interpreted broadly as meaning "a state of complete physical, mental and social wellbeing, and not merely the absence of disease or infirmity". Evidently, basic needs, primary health care, and food and nutrition planning all have similar and complementary objectives, with somewhat different sectoral emphases. Broadly, basic needs links primarily to development policy, primary health care to health policy. "Nutrition" policy – that is, the set of actions that explicitly includes nutritional objectives – is a subset of these.

The achievement of nutritional objectives is dependent on both development and health policy (e.g., ref. *23, 24*). Moreover, health and nutrition programmes or services alone do not provide long-term solutions to nutritional problems (*2*, p. 25). These considerations, we suggest, are leading to some consensus on strategy. This strategy essentially seeks (*a*) to enhance the nutritional effects of development policies and programmes that are already occurring or being planned for primarily economic and political reasons; (*b*) to rationalize and carry out effectively specific targeted programmes in the conventional nutrition and health fields; and (*c*) to prevent short-term critical reductions in food consumption. Support for such a strategy is the main *raison d'être* of nutritional surveillance. The need to define clearly the series of measures – we suggest within such a framework – is urgent (*2*, p. 20). The next two sections briefly review the relation of this strategy to policies concerned with development and health, upon which it must ultimately depend.

Planning for basic needs and nutrition

The relevance of nutrition issues to overall economic strategy needs to be considered in setting the context for nutritional surveillance. This section begins with a brief historical sketch of planning and development experience – how this has led to an emphasis on planning for basic needs as well as economic growth, and the relationship between nutritional concerns and basic needs are topics that are developed later.

Attempts at comprehensive state planning during peacetime began earlier this century in the Soviet Union, and incomplete versions of such planning spread rapidly in poorer countries after the Second World War. The newly independent nations wanted to accelerate their economic growth and thought the best way of doing this would be through the planning of investments favouring industry. Agriculture – thought of as unresponsive to prices, traditional, and facing low international prices – was to be taxed and the surplus was somehow to be transferred to the dynamic manufacturing sector. The need for foreign exchange was to be reduced through import substitution, and high rates of saving and investment in industry were to spark rapid growth.

There was a major role for government in this, both ideologically and in fact. Taxation and direction of subsidies require bureaucracies. It was initially thought that apolitical engineers and economists would select the best investments based on technical criteria. This was not so in practice. Planning is an intensely political process. It reflects not only national value judgements and strategies, but also competing interest groups trying to mobilize resources for their own special programmes. Private interests, regional groups, and coalitions within the bureaucracy all vie for a given budget. The final result is inevitably a compromise embodying ideology, idealism, technical realities, and parochial politics. In this arena, nutrition and health objectives have tended to take low priority.

The economic results of such strategies have themselves been mixed. Economic growth rates were often accelerated in average terms – certainly in market economy countries – frequently at the expense of greatly reduced impact on poverty, and even deleterious effects on income distribution. The bias towards concentrated and capital-intensive industrialization resulted in low prices for agriculture. Low prices meant little growth in output for the rural population, and governments soon realized that a stagnant agricultural sector would ruin the chances of sustained growth. Rather than raise farm prices to world levels – which could have combated this trend – most governments decided to subsidize inputs. They provided research and advice, and subsidized fertilizers, irrigation, and access to low-cost credit, and sometimes machinery. Not surprisingly, these subsidies often helped the larger and more commercially-oriented farmers more than they did the smaller farmers or landless labourers. The development of import-substituting industries has not generated much new employment in spite of adequate economic growth overall, because it has resulted in little shift in employment patterns to favour the poor. National planning thus began by discriminating against agriculture, and hence in rural areas, where the majority of the poor live, brought little improvement in the lot of the poor. One solution proposed was to plan not only for growth, but also for basic human needs.

Planning for basic human needs means planning for universal availability, at levels adequate to meet minimum needs, of food, clothing, shelter, and social services (10, 22). This partially overlaps with food and nutrition planning and also goes beyond it: basic needs include housing and education, which food and nutrition planning does not; food and nutrition planning is concerned with the export and import, processing, and marketing of food that may relate more to overall growth than to basic needs. Both types of planning have turned out to be difficult to implement. Planning for industry or large-scale agriculture involves vocal interest groups that can effectively communicate problems to adminis-trators. But there is no well organized, domestic interest group for basic needs or nutrition. No single ministry sees it as being a central focus of activity. It has evolved more as an organizational concept than as a clear-cut field for invest-ment. The lack of interest groups, of a forceful institutional base, and of a well-defined investment programme has resulted in slow progress. The outlook continues clouded as well, as renewed concern with growth, foreign exchange, and political issues shifts attention away from a still ill-defined problem, and still farther away from any obvious set of solutions. These considerations have set limits to the possible contributions of basic needs and consideration of nutritional issues in planning. Planning can only help governments efficiently realize their goals, not change strong underlying preferences. Yet a clear definition of a problem, a suggestion of its severity, and a plan for action may persuade some decision-makers that remedial measures are feasible. This feasibility, in turn, depends on the overall development strategy. Here again, there is a clear potential role for nutritional surveillance.

Health strategies

Until perhaps the early 1970s, the place of nutrition in health strategies was straightforward. Malnutrition was widely seen as a medical problem and health-related solutions were considered appropriate. Malnutrition was also regarded as stemming from ignorance – it was believed that if only mothers knew how to feed their children, their resources would be adequate for them to do so: taboos against protein foods gained wide exposure. Both protein foods and nutrition education could be delivered through the health system.

Protein lack, whether due to ignorance or supply factors, was regarded as the major nutrient supply and consumption problem and kwashiorkor was seen as the major macronutrient deficiency syndrome. The more prevalent, but medi-cally less dramatic marasmus received less attention. This causality – protein and ignorance – was appealingly soluble: close the protein gap and educate mothers. As we know now, this view of causality was based on inadequate data and knowledge (see e.g., ref. 25). In 1972, a Joint FAO/WHO Expert Committee (26) reconsidered the protein requirements, and it became clear that adequate intakes of traditional diets (in terms of energy) could almost always provide enough protein (anyway when based on cereals, which account for more than 90% of the staple diet in developing countries (see ref. 27, Appendix J8)).

The effects of infection on nutrition have been recognized for much of the same period (see ref. 28). Sick children's nutritional status deteriorates – they fail to grow or they waste – owing to anorexia, malabsorption, and the catabolic effects of infection. Adults become debilitated through biological mechanisms and because sickness reduces earning capacity and productivity, and hence purchasing power and food consumption.

Good health and good nutritional status are thus totally interdependent. Enough food is needed for good health; freedom from disease is needed for good nutritional status. This interdependence is crucial for intervention, whether health or nutritional status is the main objective, and these objectives are nearly the same: adequate preventive and curative health measures are of themselves essential for good nutrition; access to adequate food is essential for good health. This interdependence is important to concepts of primary health care, adequate nutrition being one target of primary health care strategies (15, p. 53). The relation has been further developed by a WHO Expert Committee on the Role of the Health Sector in Food and Nutrition (2). This group went so far as to propose that "food for all" was essential to achieving health for all – which is undoubtedly true.

"Primary health care entails basically a health concept and a development strategy" (2, p. 19-20). Health for all thus requires wide-ranging improvements not only in access to medical services, but parallel social and economic developments. Health services have developed with a lopsided focus on curative, high-technology, urbanized medicine. Their distribution is not equitably related to need (2, p. 16). The choices are painfully real: "... each dollar spent in Latin America on highly specialized hospital services costs a hundred lives... had each dollar been spent on providing safe drinking water and in supplying food to the population, a hundred lives could have been saved..." (de Ahumade quoted in ref. 29, p. 28); even if there is some exaggeration, the principle is correct.

Decentralization and broadening the base are the themes of the WHO strategy for health for all. This orientation promises advances in nutritional status and provides an important role for nutritional information in the policy-making, planning, and programming for primary health care.

For much of this book, nutritional and health objectives are regarded as interchangeable. This is in line with the fact that nutritional outcome indicators, as used in nutritional surveillance, are essentially the same as those for defining health outcome. Specifically, national health status indicators as defined by WHO (13, p. 18) are:

- nutritional status and psychosocial development of children;
- infant mortality rate;
- child mortality rate (ages 1-4 years inclusive);
- life expectancy at birth or other specific ages;
- maternal mortality rate.

In nutritional surveillance, the most common indicators as defined in *Nutrition in preventive medicine* (*50*) are:
- nutritional status of preschool children;
- infant and child mortality rates;
- prevalence of low birth weight;
- height of children at school entry.

Nutritional and related data thus provide core information for developing health systems and for introducing nutritional and health concerns into other sectors. Because nutrition is recognized as the concern of other sectors, it provides a useful link with them. But in the health sector itself, planning or country health programming (*14*, p. 21) depends on such data for defining problems, targeting, and deciding on causes and feasible interventions.

For monitoring progress towards health objectives and evaluation of outcome, similar indicators are needed on a regular basis. Here again, nutritional indicators and the systems that provide these are a central part of the recommended health information (*13*, p. 32). Specifically, the indicators for use by countries have been categorized as follows (*13*, p. 18):
- health policy indicators;
- social and economic indicators related to health;
- indicators of the provision of health care;
- health status indicators.

Nutritional surveillance covers most of these health indicators and provides proxies for many social and economic indicators related to health.

Finally, it must be emphasized that health information systems and nutritional surveillance systems are themselves interdependent. Most nutritional surveillance systems reach outside the health sector in two ways. The decisions based on the data, usually mediated through intersectoral coordinating bodies, relate to resource allocations, policies, and programme designs, particularly in economic planning, agriculture, and social welfare, as well as health. Secondly, core data are usually derived from the health sector, but almost invariably socioeconomic information comes from other sources.

Since adequate nutrition is a prerequisite of "health for all", policies for nutrition must become a concern of the advocates of health for all. The health sector alone cannot do everything needed to ensure good nutrition, and this implies the need for substantial intersectoral cooperation, for it is rare that the health sector has a lot of direct influence on the activities of ministries who can affect food availability to malnourished families. While individual welfare is the main objective of the health sector, this is often not true of other sectors such as agriculture, which are primarily concerned with aggregate production. This means, in effect, that in so far as pressure for action to ensure health for all can be used to promote progress towards good nutrition (as a prerequisite for health for all), this must come from a higher political level than the ministry of health; it must in fact come from the realization that adequate health and nutrition are national objectives that need to be achieved by the activities of a number of different sectors. The health sector can contribute to reaching this objective: first, by making the problems clear, and secondly by helping to produce the information to support this. Further, it is logical that a part of the resources necessary for achieving "health for all" would need to be used in at least planning and monitoring progress towards adequate nutrition. This means that commitment to a "health for all" objective includes, among other things, support for nutritional surveillance.

Relation of health, nutrition, and basic needs to different national development strategies

Different national development strategies imply different roles for health, nutrition, and basic needs objectives in national planning. Three types of strategy are suggested in Table 1.2 with quite different circumstances and governmental goals. The format leaves out a number of cases – the richer developing countries do not easily fit into it, nor do those countries, both rich and poor, that put little emphasis on ameliorating poverty. None the less, the three types discussed open up a fairly rich set of opportunities for health, nutrition, and basic needs objectives in national planning.

In general, if asset redistribution is combined with a sustained, moderate to rapid rate of economic growth, there are unlikely to be major health and nutritional problems springing from chronic poverty (see subtype 1A in Table 1.2). Certain geographical regions may be isolated – backward, poor, and subject to large fluctuations in crop output. Investments in infrastructure or output-stabilizing techniques may be required in such cases. Vulnerable groups (i.e., young children and pregnant or lactating mothers) may well need additional services. In each case, the problem is often evident and already reflected in a national plan of action.

The second subtype (1B) differs in several ways from the first. The resources redistributed are of income available to the government from production, rather than productive assets themselves. Since assets have not been redistributed, there is a need to rely on transfer payments to a greater extent. This can result in low investment and growth rates, which slow the general increase in incomes. It can also lead to a reaction against the transfer payments as the middle-income groups become impatient with slow progress and connect it with an unsatisfactory trade-off between investment and welfare. Considerations of health and nutritional needs can help to target services and income transfers to make them more efficient.

Table 1.2. Typology of development strategies and the role of nutrition and basic needs in national planning [a]

Type	Strategy	Characteristics	Role of nutrition and basic needs in planning	Examples of countries in each category
1A	Asset redistribution	Initially poor; moderate–fast growth; prices "realistic"	Small–supportive	China, Republic of Korea
1B	Natural resource rents for social welfare	Political competition; investment vs. welfare trade-offs; slow–medium growth	Moderate within overall basic needs framework	Jamaica, Sri Lanka
2	Capitalist growth with inequality (but social services provided)	High *per capita* GNP; high urbanization; high inequality; high capacity for social service delivery	Moderate but restricted	Chile, Colombia
3	Mixed – mainly growth with secondary basic needs concern	Low–middle income and urbanization; limited intervention capacity	Potentially high	Indonesia, Kenya

[a] This table draws heavily on J.O. Field's paper, *The importance of context: nutrition planning and development reconsidered* (19). However, the typology used is somewhat different from his.

Perhaps the major point is that in the asset and rent redistribution types (1A and 1B of Table 1.2) of development strategy the reduction of poverty and the ability to improve government administration through political processes or better management make significant progress in health and nutrition relatively easy and natural. Planning for basic needs, primary health care, and nutrition continues what has already been well begun. It can help identify those people most needing attention and evaluate the effectiveness of remedial efforts, and is basically supported by the major thrust of governmental policies.

In the second, quite different type of situation (2 in Table 1.2) direct interventions to alleviate the effects of poverty are seen as marginal to the main thrust of economic strategy. Governments adopting this strategy are willing to let time and income growth deal with the structural causes of poverty, but wish to reduce the effects of it via programmes aimed at improving health and nutrition. These programmes will be mainly for vulnerable groups and may include targeted small food subsidies. Since income per capita is comparatively high, the relatively low cost of the programmes need not put too much strain on government budgets, and the high urbanization rate facilitates easy access to many of the poor. Fairly good administration and adequate supplies of skilled personnel make the initiatives easier as well. Nutritional objectives in this case can be useful in directing these efforts, but are clearly confined to the programmes themselves. The relatively low infant mortality rates in Colombia and Chile, for example, compared with Brazil suggest that such programmes can have an impact under these conditions.

The third type of development strategy (3 in Table 1.2) is probably typical of more countries than the others. Most developing countries have relatively low incomes, modest levels of urbanization (especially outside of Latin America), and limited supplies of skilled personnel. Few of these countries are able or willing to redistribute assets or have enough rent to change drastically the consumption patterns and services for the poor. For this group, poverty has to be tackled through the growth process, but with less than radical change. This means raising and stabilizing the output and consumption of the poor, most of whom will be farmers or farm labourers. Many of the necessary steps on the output side are familiar in the context of "integrated rural development": appropriate technologies, agricultural advisory services, available credit, help with "lumpy" inputs such as irrigation or some machinery, and supportive pricing policies are all needed. Bottlenecks in processing, storing, or marketing of food often have to be tackled, especially if private markets are sluggish or unable to handle some of the larger infrastructure. Social services of a very basic kind will also be required.

It is in the context of these latter development strategies that considerations of nutrition, basic needs, and primary health care are particularly required. This is because, in contrast to the others, improvements in health, nutrition, and basic needs cannot be assumed to come about as a result of existing policies and programmes. These countries, generally relatively poor and going for growth rather than distribution, do not have the resources for large-scale welfare programmes and rapid expansion of services. Their main option for tackling poverty and its effects is an ability to direct investment to a greater or lesser extent. Decisions on this require careful planning and difficult trade-offs. How far these decisions actually favour health, nutrition, and basic needs depends on the political interactions discussed earlier – interest groups, institutional base, and so on – but also requires a knowledge of the problems, their causes, and how they are changing. Nutritional surveillance provides an essential part of this knowledge.

Actions to Improve Nutrition and Related Data Requirements

Logically, defining the actions required to alleviate malnutrition should start with an analysis of the problem, followed by setting objectives, analysing policy instruments for reaching these objectives, and finally selecting the appropriate instruments. Although this procedure is seldom followed faithfully in practice, it provides a starting point.

Some policy commitment on the part of the government to promoting good nutrition is a prerequisite for deciding on and implementing the necessary actions. How far nutritional surveillance itself can initiate such policy decisions is not well known. It has been claimed that the purpose of nutritional surveillance is part of a continuing attempt to change government policy in favour of nutrition or social equity, where such concerns are missing.[1] We have not found any examples of actual surveillance activities that are achieving this purpose – probably because it is unlikely that the ongoing character of nutritional surveillance can be established in the face of a governmental policy that is unconcerned with nutrition and social equity. This may be contrasted with the usefulness of short-term nutritional assessment endeavours that do not require long-term commitments, can be accomplished in spite of a lack of governmental interest, and can indeed on occasions change policy. On the other hand, surveillance data can in theory reinforce public and governmental policy in favour of better nutrition and more social equity – but some interest must already exist to initiate nutritional surveillance. In our opinion, the more fruitful view of nutritional surveillance is that it follows some governmental policy commitment to nutritional objectives.

Once a policy commitment is made – even if only in rather general terms at the outset – options must be identified and subsequently selected to further that policy. The purposes of nutritional surveillance can be to facilitate the choice of these options, the design of the actions themselves, their evaluation, and on

---

[1] *Report of the International Workshop on Nutritional Surveillance held in Cali, Colombia, 14-19 July, 1981,* Rome, ACC-SCN, 1982 (document SCN 82/10).

Table 1.3. Policies and programmes affecting nutrition

Policy or programme	Relevance of information from nutritional surveillance
National policies, e.g.: — resource allocations, by area and sector — legislative: e.g., price policy, commodity flows, minimum wages. — programme directions: e.g., promoting different crops — preventive/curative health measures	Planning
Development programmes, e.g.: — area development programmes — commodity programmes	Planning and evaluation
Public health and nutrition programmes, e.g.: — environmental health — primary health care	Planning and evaluation
Timely warning and intervention programmes — for famine prevention — for alleviating seasonal food shortages	Initiating interventions

occasion (e.g., timely warning) to give notice that special measures must be initiated. Reviewing briefly these options is the next step that is necessary for understanding the role of nutritional surveillance (see Table 1.3). Many actions could be used to affect nutrition: broadly, these fall into the categories of programmes and of legislative measures that are not implemented through programmes in the usual sense (sometimes themselves referred to as "policies"). Programmes guide the activities of government or other personnel and provide the goods and services for these activities, e.g., health programmes, agricultural programmes. Legislative measures, such as setting the prices paid to producers, or charged to consumers, regulating the flow of commodities, or setting minimum wages are not generally carried out through programmes in the same sense but clearly may require substantial resources and can have crucial effects on nutrition. Decisions in both these areas are discussed below under the heading "Inputs to national policies".

Secondly, the design, management, and evaluation of individual programmes – particularly in health and development – may offer opportunities for alleviating malnutrition. The issues here are often more easily identified. Rural development programmes and nutrition and health programmes are discussed below.

Finally, prevention of short-term food consumption crises raises other issues still – of particular relevance to nutritional surveillance – and the types of programmes needed to deal with these are referred to as "timely warning and intervention programmes".

In laying out the different possibilities for tackling nutrition problems, emphasis is given to the methods for deciding on and planning the appropriate measures, and to the respective data requirements.

Inputs to national policies

A fundamental set of decisions in national planning concerns the allocation of resources between administrative regions and different activities (e.g., by sector) affecting different socioeconomic groups. These allocations determine how far resources are directed toward the malnourished; and knowledge of the relative needs of different groups – in geographical and socioeconomic terms – can be used to recommend attention to the malnourished. These decisions are often made first in the context of national development plans, usually five-yearly with annual revisions. A procedure for reviewing these plans in relation to their relevance to nutrition requires institutional links (e.g., nutrition units in planning ministries), analytical methods, and data.

Then there are major policy goals within which decisions will necessarily affect nutrition: self-sufficiency in food is one example, with its associated choices to do with agricultural development, pricing, and so on. Different ways of reaching this goal can have profoundly different effects on health, nutrition, and basic needs. For example, similar production targets might be reached either through capital-intensive irrigated agriculture or through extensive rain-fed production by smallholders: yet these choices are seldom reviewed in the light of their likely effects on the needy. Two practical issues in national policy-making, often seen in the context of self-sufficiency, are discussed in more detail for illustration: the pricing of staple foods and the choice between cash crops and food crops.

Attention has been increasingly focused in the last few years on the possibility of manipulating food prices as a means of increasing the food consumption of the poor, as well as of increasing supply (e.g., ref. 31). Indeed, this has been described as possibly being "the only financially feasible way of coping with protein-calorie malnutrition over the next several decades" (31, p. 199). Administrative targeting of food subsidy schemes (as opposed to targeting by selection of commodity, e.g., less-preferred foods for the poor) using food stamps, etc., is one possible means of increasing efficiency, but such methods face serious administrative constraints in many countries. Pricing major grains is typically a highly political issue. There are many dimensions to the decisions: rich–poor, urban–rural, and often regional. These decisions often have major influences on production, imports, consumption, and the government budget. None the less, politically acceptable possibilities exist for improving the consumption of the malnourished. For example, if different regions or socioeconomic groups eat different staples, it may be possible to lower the price of one staple while raising that of another so that consumers who can easily make substitutions (often the poor) can swap high-cost ''energy'', such as from rice, for low-cost energy from other staples. Nutritional and dietary information can support this type of analysis, as well as providing for assessment of the overall impact on aggregate consumption, production, and trade.

The issue of cash crops versus food crops is another that troubles many governments. Since food is a basic need, it is plausible that not too much should depend on foreign supply. Yet often there is a substantial sacrifice in income if specialization is ignored. Some observations suggest that nutrition may worsen even while incomes increase if farmers shift from a subsistence to a cash crop (particularly export crop) system. How does a policy-maker balance these issues and reach a reasonable decision? Nutritional surveillance can make a contribution by indicating whether malnutrition does in fact increase as a shift is made from subsistence to cash crops. Observation of vulnerable groups in different areas may also suggest whether certain crops, cultures, or conditions give rise to especially high risks, and may point towards remedial activities. Here again, nutritional information may allow prediction and prevention of negative side-effects of agricultural policies.

In designing programmes at national level – either national programmes themselves or the distribution of area-specific programmes – two of the basic issues are targeting and choosing programme options for those targeted. Certain programmes, such as in health, are targeted mainly by administrative area. Others, as in agricultural or rural development, are targeted in fact both by area and by socioeconomic group, defined by occupation, farming pattern, land-holding size, and tenure, etc. – for example, agricultural inputs may be focused on certain crops or on farmers with a minimum land-holding. Nutritional data can be used for both targeting and choosing programme options, but are particularly suitable for targeting. Choosing among the different types of programmes – the more so when nutritional benefit is an objective – requires more extensive information. Programme design choices, for example, which commodities to produce, or preventive *versus* curative health, are made as part of national policy; more detailed design choices for individual programmes are discussed in the next section.

The methods for introducing nutritional considerations into national planning need brief consideration, since these determine the data requirements and hence the specific role of nutritional surveillance for these purposes. They also have relevance to the programme planning described in the next section. Broadly, two methods can be applied to the assessment of the nutritional implications of national policies. First, a functional classification can be structured to provide a framework for examining the relevance of policies to identified nutritional problems (*32, 33*). Secondly, food supply and demand projections can be analysed for their food intake implications using econometric techniques (e.g., see ref. *34*).

A functional or socioeconomic classification means essentially breaking down the population of a country into defined groups that may have different risks or prevalences of malnutrition; the nutritionally worst-off would then merit priority in benefiting from government policies, if these policies are to have a direct impact on nutrition. The main purposes of constructing such a classification are to promote targeting (and also an analysis of the outreach of existing policies) and to gain certain insights into the causes of malnutrition and hence possible solutions. Only a very few countries have yet completed a classification of their populations in this way (e.g., ref. *35*), although the elements of this type of thinking are familiar – for instance, in certain approaches to economic development planning (*36*). However, in a number of countries where the information is available and suitable institutions exist, steps are being taken in this direction.

Building up this type of framework – defining who is malnourished in terms relevant to economic or health planning – requires data on nutritional conditions that can be disaggregated by geographical and socioeconomic criteria. This procedure is recommended in reference *13*(p. 20, para 43). For definition of the extent of nutritional problems specific surveys may be required. Data from socioeconomic surveys and censuses can then be used to study possible solutions. Food consumption data can be used when available to classify functional groups nutritionally, but it is usually more feasible to use nutritional status and health indicators. Evidently, following changes in such indicators would amount to nutritional surveillance at national level.

Projections of food supply and demand have become routine in many countries in the context of national development plans. The implications of these projections in relation to nutritional requirements (usually in terms of energy) can be quite readily calculated, at least in average terms. These calculations almost invariably show that without significant redistribution of income, the projected changes in effective demand of low-income groups will be insufficient to provide for the rates of change in food consumption necessary to meet their nutritional requirements within a reasonable time period – the same conclusions as reached at more aggregate level (see, for example, ref. *27, 37, 38*). Moreover, in most cases, at least in the medium term, the inadequate effective demand of the poor is more of a constraint to their food consumption than overall food supply. This type of approach has been extended to mathematical modelling of national economies e.g., in Iran,[1] and in Pakistan (*39*). Comprehensive data systems and related methods are also proposed (*36, 40*), and used for analysis in some cases (e.g., ref. *41*).

Projections of food supply and demand require detailed production, income/expenditure, and consumption data, obtained from agricultural and household budget surveys. These surveys are at present usually carried out on a one-time

---

[1] PYATT, G.F. ET AL. *Employment and income policies for Iran: methodology for macro-economic projection. Comprehensive Employment Strategy Mission to Iran, Working Paper No. 12,* Geneva, International Labour Office, 1973 (unpublished document).

basis, and are expensive; they do not need to be established on a continuing basis, although obtaining such data could be an important function of ongoing survey systems if these were sufficiently well developed. Data requirements for analysis of price effects are more demanding – for example, in sample size, the extent of the data needed for sample households, and the desirability of time-series data. Detailed analyses have been attempted in only a few countries, e.g., Colombia (42), Indonesia (31), and Pakistan (39). The large-scale Indonesian socioeconomic survey, with 54 000 households in three rounds, was just adequate to permit the required analysis for certain commodities. This scale and type of data collection may also be better carried out on a one-time basis, if only because of the resources needed. While the purpose of nutritional surveillance may not be to provide data to support price-policy analysis itself, tracing the effects of price policies on nutritional conditions in the country concerned could be an important function of a nutritional surveillance system.

Inputs to programme planning and management

Development programmes

Many of the resources currently allocated to development are provided through programmes; that is, they are confined geographically, in time, and to a determined set of activities or components. In many cases foreign funds, such as loans or grants, are used to cover part of the costs, particularly in the form of foreign exchange. In some countries, this often means that in practice the donor agencies do much of the programme planning and frequently influence implementation. Such programmes are the main vehicle for development assistance from donor agencies, both multinational and bilateral. Programmes may be oriented to single sectors or commodities or may be more general and multi-component in nature. In many countries, donors are assigned to different regions, and the area development programmes subsequently prepared and implemented in these regions are becoming a major channel for government and foreign funds.

Rural or area development programmes, in particular, frequently include as stated objectives improvements in the quality of life, satisfaction of basic needs, etc. These programmes are also of special interest in the context of nutrition because, given enough resources, and no preconceptions or sectoral constraints, designing a project to bring about long-term improvement in nutrition would result in something that closely resembles a conventional rural or area development project.

In theory, the design issues and the data needs for planning development programmes are similar to those for national planning. In practice, there are important differences. First, data on production, income, etc., may be available from national surveys, but can seldom be validly disaggregated to apply to programme areas. Further, a "food balance sheet" approach cannot usually be used since trade into and out of the area is not known. Thus, special-purpose surveys may be required, although the limited resources available for programme planning may often preclude detailed survey work. Second, it may be easier to link together planning, monitoring, and evaluation at the level of a programme; and indeed there may be more interest in doing this.

The simplest approach to assessing the nutritional effects of development programmes, and to monitoring these, is to start by addressing the questions "who benefits from the project – in relation to their degree of nutritional deprivation?" and "will the programme improve the nutrition of those who participate?" (5). Outcome data analysed by socioeconomic group are the main requirements for answering these questions.[1] Repeated collection of these variables would allow monitoring of actual outcome for evaluation. The next level of approach involves projecting changes in food consumption, from the anticipated income increases resulting from the project and possibly from postulated price effects (43). This method requires production/income/consumption data at programme area level.

Health and nutrition programmes and services

Health and nutrition programmes and services conventionally include: public health measures, such as water supply, sanitation, immunization, health service, and health education; and nutritional interventions, such as supplementary feeding, rehabilitation, nutrition education, fortification, and enrichment of foods. Many of these programmes are operated through the health system and form the core of primary health care. Their planning and implementation is thus frequently the responsibility of ministries of health, organized through area offices, health posts and clinics. Certain of these activities may be included as components of development programmes. Infrastructure development – including water supply as a prime example – can obviously have a profound direct effect on the health environment, and a less direct effect, for example, by facilitating access (e.g., by road-building) to health services. Nutrition programmes have a wider, but perhaps less committed, institutional base in many countries. While many such programmes are operated by the health sector, those concerned with food distribution in particular may fall under other ministries, including agriculture, local government, and education. Also, several countries have established national nutrition agencies; however, the activities of these usually still depend on the traditional government agencies (notably health and agriculture), and their role is substantially a coordinating one, except when they channel extensive funds (as in certain Latin American countries).

---

[1] GARCIA, M.H. *Palawan case study*. Manila, National Nutrition Council, 1980 (unpublished document); MASON, J.B. *Case study for FAO on introducing nutrition considerations into development project planning – Haiti*. Ithaca, NY, Cornell University, 1980 (unpublished document).

International aid for health programmes is given by most donor agencies – often linked with population and nutrition activities. Within the United Nations system, WHO is the leading agency in this field. UNICEF also provides funds for many health programmes. As is the case nationally, international support for nutrition programmes is also diffuse. In the United Nations, coordinating responsibility is with the Administrative Committee on Coordination – Sub-Committee on Nutrition (ACC-SCN). UNICEF, FAO, WHO and the World Bank all have certain responsibilities for these programmes – FAO and WHO, largely with their counterpart ministries of agriculture and health, respectively. UNICEF supports programmes in cooperation with a variety of government agencies, as do a substantial number of volunteer organizations.

Present opinion on the role of public health and nutrition programmes in tackling malnutrition takes several positions, reflecting in part an inadequate knowledge of the effectiveness of these programmes. The support for decentralized health care services is well established, as is that for such mainstays of preventive medicine as immunization, and water supply and sanitation. Nutrition programmes have a less well-established role. There is evidence to indicate that their impact has been disappointing, according to a WHO Expert Committee (2) because of: "(1) Inadequate coverage of the population by health care services, the groups in greatest need having the poorest services, if any at all. Nutrition measures, through the health sector, therefore hardly reach this segment. (2) Adoption of nutrition interventions which were either inappropriate or unadaptable to the local conditions". Only relatively recently have careful comparative evaluations for a range of programmes become available (e.g., ref. 44-46). Broadly, the conclusions from these evaluations are that some impact is found when health and nutrition activities are combined, but that the evidence for nutrition interventions having an effect in isolation is scanty. This may, in part, reflect poor design and management of nutrition interventions; greater attention to the relevance and feasibility of such interventions is, therefore, needed at the design stage.[1] Furthermore, the level of resources applied is often not sufficient, with implementation deviating significantly from that planned, to expect that any wide effect will be detected on evaluation (47, 48).

Design of health and nutrition programmes needs to take account of targeting and appropriateness of possible programme options if the problem is to be tackled successfully. Their management requires data to evaluate the process of implementation and the outcome, in relation to programme objectives (15). These data can also be used for deciding about future programmes, and for deciding on extension, modification or ending of the programme being

---

[1] BEGHIN, I. *Selection of specific nutritional components for agricultural and rural development projects.* Antwerp, Institute of Tropical Medicine, 1980 (unpublished document).

evaluated. The data required are therefore similar to those for other purposes, but additionally require information on programme delivery. Methods for routine evaluation for management are in need of further clarification, and suggestions for this are presented in Chapter 5.

Timely warning and intervention programmes

In some situations major episodes of malnutrition are brought about by relatively short-term events – imposed on conditions of severe poverty – such as drought, crop damage, pests, price changes for agricultural products, and, certainly, conflicts and wars. It may also be that for certain people experiencing intermittent poor harvests leading to acute but transient food shortages of less than famine scale, specific measures to combat these could be important in long-term alleviation of chronic malnutrition. Chronic malnutrition, which is much the larger problem numerically, could thus be helped by preventing repeated acute episodes. A series of interventions can be planned to forestall the nutritional effects of some of these events. Information on impending problems must trigger such interventions in good time. In such situations, interventions and information are closely linked, as far as possible in a predetermined way, and can be called "timely warning and intervention programmes" (TWIPs). Experience has shown that only in particular circumstances do such programmes get off the ground – and that they have distinct resource, organizational, and data needs that are different from those of either planning or evaluation. This is not to say that timely warning and intervention cannot be a part of a more general nutritional surveillance programme. However, its purposes and requirements are sufficiently different to merit discussion in their own right. "Timely warning" has in the past been known as "early warning". This has caused some misunderstanding: the timing of the warning relates only to the lead time needed to launch an effective intervention. The warning must be linked administratively to triggering the intervention, and needs to be no earlier than this. Hence we have adopted the term "timely warning and intervention programme".

The type of data needed to provide timely warning of possible food consumption crises depends on the likely causes. If the causes are primarily related to food crop failure, then early estimates of production are likely to be needed. When the causes of deteriorating consumption are due to fall in demand, other indicators, such as levels of employment, may be needed. Later in the sequence of events, price data may provide evidence of change, and later still, health and nutrition indicators will reflect the consequences of decreasing food consumption. Further discussion of timely warning and intervention is presented in Chapter 6.

REFERENCES

1. *Alma-Ata 1978: Primary health care*. Geneva, World Health Organization, 1978 ("Health for All" Series, No. 2).

2. WHO Technical Report Series, No. 667, 1981 (*The role of the health sector in food and nutrition. Report of a WHO Expert Committee*).

3. *Report of the World Food Conference, Rome, 5-6 November 1974*. New York, United Nations, 1975 (Publication E/Conf. 65/20).

4. WHO Technical Report Series, No. 593, 1976 (*Methodology of nutritional surveillance. Report of a Joint FAO/UNICEF/WHO Expert Committee*).

5. *Nutrition in Agriculture. Fifth Session of the Committee on Agriculture*. Rome, Food and Agriculture Organization of the United Nations, 1979 (LOAG 7916).

6. FOEGE, W. H. ET AL. Surveillance projects for selected diseases. *International journal of epidemiology*, **5**: 29-37 (1976).

7. LWANGA, S. Statistical principles of monitoring and surveillance in public health. *Bulletin of the World Health Organization*, **56**: 713-722 (1978).

8. NICHAMAN, M. Z. Developing a nutritional surveillance system. *Journal of the American Dietetic Association*, **65**: 15-17 (1974).

9. MASON, J. B. ET AL. Nutritional lessons from the Ethiopian drought. *Nature (London)*, **248**: 646-650 (1974).

10. *Meeting basic needs. Strategies for eradicating mass poverty and unemployment*, Geneva, International Labour Office, 1977.

11. CASLEY, D. J. & LURY, D. A. *A handbook on monitoring and evaluation of agricultural and rural development projects*. Washington, DC, World Bank, 1981.

12. *Health programme evaluation: Guiding principles*. Geneva, World Health Organization, 1981 ("Health for All" Series, No. 6).

13. *Development of indicators for monitoring progress towards health for all by the year 2000*. Geneva, World Health Organization, 1981 ("Health for All" Series, No. 4).

14. *Formulating strategies for health for all by the year 2000*. Geneva, World Health Organization, 1979 ("Health for All" Series, No. 2).

15. *Global strategy for health for all by the year 2000*. Geneva, World Health Organization, 1981 ("Health for All" Series, No. 3).

16. JONSSON, U. The causes of hunger. *Food and nutrition bulletin*, **3**: 1-9 (1981).

17. WHO Technical Report Series, No. 584, 1976 (*Food and nutrition strategies in national development. Ninth report of the Joint FAO/WHO Expert Committee on Nutrition*).

18. TAYLOR, L. The misconstrued crisis: Lester Brown and world food. *World development*, **3**: 827-837 (1975).

19. FIELD, J. O. The importance of context: Nutrition planning and development reconsidered. In: McLaren, D. S., ed. *Nutrition in the community*, 2nd ed. Chichester, Wiley, 1983.

20. FIELD, J. O. The soft underbelly of applied knowledge. Conceptual and operational problems in nutrition planning. *Food policy*, **2** (3): 228-239 (1977).

21. LYNCH, L. Nutrition planning methodologies: A comparative review of types and applications. *Food and nutrition bulletin*, **1**: 1-14 (1979).

22. *Employment, growth and basic needs. A one-world problem*. Geneva, International Labour Office, 1976.

23. MELLOR, J. W. Nutrition and economic growth. In: Berg, A. et al., *Nutrition, national development and planning*, Cambridge, MIT Press, 1973, pp. 70-73.

24. LATHAM, M. C. Strategies to control infections in malnourished populations – holistic approach or narrowly targeted interventions? *American journal of clinical nutrition,* **31**: 2292-2300 (1978).

25. McLAREN, D. S. The great protein fiasco. *Lancet,* **2**: 93-96 (1974).

26. WHO Technical Report Series, No. 522, 1973 *(Energy and protein requirements. Report of a Joint FAO/WHO Ad Hoc Expert Committee).*

27. FAO Statistics Series, No. 11; FAO Food and Nutrition Series, No. 10, 1977 *(The fourth world food survey).*

28. SCRIMSHAW, N. S. ET AL. *Interactions of nutrition and infection.* Geneva, World Health Organization, 1968 (WHO Monograph Series, No. 57).

29. NAVARRO, V. The underdevelopment of health or the health of underdevelopment: an analysis of the distribution of human health resources in Latin America. In: Navarro, V., ed. *Imperialism, health and medicine,* Farmingdale, NY, Baywood Publishing Co., 1981, pp. 15-36.

30. Fourth Latin American Nutrition Congress: Colloquium on Nutritional Epidemiological Surveillance Systems. *Archivos Latinoamericános de nutrición,* **27** (2), Suppl. 1, June 1977.

31. TIMMER, C. P. Food prices and food policy analysis in LDCs. *Food policy,* **5** (3): 188-199 (1980).

32. JOY, J. L. Food and nutrition planning. *Journal of agricultural economics,* **24:** 165-192 (1973).

33. JOY, J. L. & PAYNE, P. R. *Food and nutrition planning,* Rome, Food and Agriculture Organization of the United Nations, 1975 (FAO Nutrition Consultants Reports Series, No. 35).

34. PERISSE, J. The nutritional approach in food policy planning. *The FAO nutrition newsletter,* **6** (1): 30-47 (1968).

35. VALVERDE, V. ET AL. Functional classification of undernourished populations in the Republic of El Salvador. Methodological development. *Food and nutrition,* **4**: 8-14 (1978).

36. PYATT, G. F. & THORBECKE, P. *Planning for a better future.* Geneva, International Labour Office, 1976.

37. REUTLINGER, S. & SELOWSKY, M. *Malnutrition and poverty. Magnitude and policy options.* Washington, DC, World Bank (World Bank Staff Occasional Papers, No. 23).

38. REUTLINGER, S. & ALDERMAN, H. The prevalence of calorie-deficient diets in developing countries. *World development,* **8**: 399-411 (1980).

39. McCARTHY, D. & TAYLOR, L. Macro food policy planning: a general equilibrium model for Pakistan. *Review of economics and statistics,* 62: 107-121 (1980).

40. HAY, R. W. The statistics of hunger. *Food policy,* **3** (4): 243-255 (1978).

41. PYATT, G. & ROE, A. R. *Social accounting for development planning with special reference to Sri Lanka.* Cambridge, Cambridge University Press, 1977.

42. PINSTRUP-ANDERSEN, P. ET AL. The impact of increasing food supply on human nutrition: implications for commodity priorities in agricultural research and policy. *American journal of agricultural economics,* May 1976, pp. 131-142.

43. PINSTRUP-ANDERSEN, P. *Nutritional consequences of agricultural projects. Conceptual relationships and assessment approaches.* Washington, DC, World Bank, 1981 (World Bank Staff Working Paper, No. 456).

44. HABICHT, J.-P. & BUTZ, W. P. Measurement of health and nutrition effects of large-scale nutrition intervention projects. In: Klein, R. E. et al., ed. *Evaluating the impact of nutrition and health programs.* New York, Plenum Press, 1979.

45. BEATON, G. H. & GHASSEMI, H. Supplementary feeding programs for young children in developing countries. *American journal of clinical nutrition,* **35** (4 Suppl.): 863-916 (1982).

46. GWATKIN, D. R. ET AL. *Can health and nutrition interventions make a difference?* Washington, DC, Overseas Development Council, 1980 (ODC Monograph No. 13).

47. HABICHT, J.-P. ET AL. Basic concepts for design of evaluations during program implementation. In: Sahn, D. E. et al., ed. *Methods for evaluating the impact of food and nutrition programs.* Tokyo, United Nations University, (in press).

48. MASON, J. B. & HABICHT, J.-P. Stages of evaluation of on-going programs. In: Sahn, D. E. et al., ed. *Methods for evaluating the impact of food and nutrition programs.* Tokyo, United Nations University, (in press).

49. *Nutritional surveillance: a synopsis.* Washington, DC, National Academy of Sciences, 1982.

50. BEATON, G.H. & BENGOA, J.M. *Nutrition in preventive medicine. The major deficiency syndromes, epidemiology, and approaches to control.* Geneva, World Health Organization, 1976 (WHO Monograph Series, No. 62).

CHAPTER 2

Initial assessment

Summary

The initial assessment – or periodic reassessment – should lead to a design for nutritional surveillance that takes into account a number of important questions. The work-plan should indicate responsibilities assigned to each of the cooperating institutions, the necessary budgetary resources, and a schedule of activities and outputs. The issues mentioned below must also be decided initially, or re-examined when an on-going programme is reviewed.

The users of the information, and their needs for decision-making, must be clearly identified. These may be in national or local government, in programme management, or concerned with the prevention or relief of acute food shortages. The objectives of the system, and hence the priority given to serving the needs of different users, depend on the extent to which their activities can affect nutritional problems, and the latter need to be described, preferably as a baseline statement on the nutrition situation: the extent of malnutrition, who is affected, and major causes. Certain key pieces of information should be included in this statement in order to define the problems to be tackled and as a basis for discussion with potential users. Examples of possible outputs from a surveillance system, including cross-sectional analyses that could be repeated over time, and dummy tables should be produced to facilitate decisions on the objectives and form of the surveillance system. On the basis of these considerations, potential sources of data need to be identified; usually these will draw mainly on existing data-collection mechanisms, sometimes with the insertion of nutrition measurements in these. The data sources may thus include sample surveys and routine government services including censuses, for planning purposes; programme monitoring and evaluation systems and periodic small-scale surveys for programme management and evaluation; and, for timely warning and intervention, a range of possible indicators depending on the causes of acute food shortages, such as rainfall and food prices, usually collected through existing institutions.

Having reached preliminary conclusions on the objectives of the nutritional surveillance system and how it could operate, institutional arrangements must then be made for data collection, analysis, linkage to decision-making, and dissemination of information. Resource requirements must be assessed and should not be underestimated. As with the rest of the process, these decisions must be reached through discussions with all the institutions concerned. Put together, these decisions lead to a preliminary design of the surveillance system and a work-plan for its implementation.

Introduction

The first phase of setting up nutritional surveillance is of crucial importance and requires adequate time and resources. This phase could be called an initial assessment. The procedure discussed here is not very different from that outlined in *Methodology of nutritional surveillance* (see ref. *1*, sections 2 and 4.3). However, based on experience since those proposals were put forward, top priority is now given to determining who uses the information produced and for what purposes, and to making sure that there is a workable mechanism for linking information to decision-making.

Usually this initial assessment can form the first phase of a nutritional surveillance programme. Where information systems are being used already for surveillance purposes, but have not gone through such a process, it may still be worth reassessing exactly what the system is trying to achieve and whether it can do so as presently structured. In an existing system, therefore, this procedure provides for a periodic reassessment or review. The assessment should produce information that is itself useful for decision-making. The exercise can therefore be justified in its own right – even if it were decided not to proceed with surveillance.

The steps described here are not intended to be consecutive, and they may need to be repeated several times. They should lead to decisions on the following points:

- the users of nutritional surveillance information, the relevant policies and programmes, the topics on which information is required for decision-making, and thus the objectives of the surveillance system;
- the nutritional and related problems to be tackled;
- the information outputs needed, with examples of these;
- the potential sources of data;
- the institutional arrangements for data collection and analysis, administrative levels at which these are needed, links to users, resources required, and means of disseminating information;

Finally, a work-plan for initiating (or continuing) nutritional surveillance must be prepared, clearly indicating responsibilities and resources.

Certain basic principles must guide this process. Nutritional surveillance can be justified only if it leads to alleviation or prevention of malnutrition. It should never exist in isolation from action. The information must be used in support of planning efforts to improve nutrition; for evaluating programmes; or to provide timely warning followed by appropriate intervention to prevent the effects of sudden food shortages. These uses involve a more rational allocation of available resources to reduce the magnitude of nutritional problems. A fuller description of actions that can be taken to improve nutrition has been given in Chapter 1.

Initiatives for tackling the problems of nutrition, and hence for setting up nutritional surveillance, come from two main sources: from the nutrition "establishment" within a country, for example, the government, para-governmental bodies, universities, voluntary agencies, or donors; or from other parts of government (or donor agencies) less traditionally associated with nutrition, which for various reasons become concerned with basic needs, social welfare, or nutrition. Nutrition institutions have taken the initiative in promoting

or designing nutritional surveillance systems in many of the current programmes. These institutions, which exist in most countries, can play a key role in
providing expertise, staff, and other resources, both in the initial assessment and
subsequently. The risk is that they may fail to integrate surveillance activities
into the mainstream of government programmes. Initiatives originating outside
the traditional nutrition establishment, although often more vaguely formulated
with respect to nutrition, are likely to be more powerfully backed. These
initiatives may stem from the needs of large-scale social welfare or food
programmes, or from a more general concern with the effects of government
policies and programmes on nutrition. In this case, nutritional surveillance may
serve to support identified programme needs, such as targeting or evaluation. In
other circumstances still, the initial phase may be part of a broader planning
exercise. Opportunities for this may emerge with new initiatives in government
policy, for example, as a result of reviewing health priorities or food policies, or
in the course of regular planning procedures such as formulating development
plans and projects. However, it is always necessary to start with clear descriptions of the problems, the potential decisions, and hence the objectives of
nutritional surveillance.

Since the work required for an initial assessment is substantial, it can be
approached as a project in its own right – with objectives, a work plan, a budget,
and an establishment for personnel. The time required may be several months or
longer. The project may usefully include workshops to reach decisions on
various points, as well as training, data analysis, recommendations on current
decisions, etc. The outcome should be a detailed plan for establishing nutritional
surveillance.

Finally, it should be emphasized that nutritional surveillance should never be
set up to duplicate the role of other systems, e.g., health information systems.
Rather it should draw on, contribute to or often actually be part of other systems.

Defining the Objectives of a Nutritional Surveillance System

Nutritional surveillance systems with different objectives require different
designs. Experience has shown that these different objectives must be clearly
distinguished, and their priorities decided upon, during the design of the system.
Failure to do this prevents clear specification of workable procedures. The
different objectives are not entirely mutually exclusive, and some systems are
beginning to use data collected in the first instance for one purpose – planning,
for example – for other purposes such as evaluation. None the less, limitations in
economic and human resources restrict the scope of objectives that can be
envisaged at any one time.

The initial assessment procedure leads to a decision on objectives, based on
considerations of (a) the priority of problems of malnutrition, (b) the needs of

Table 2.1. Types of nutritional surveillance appropriate to different situations

Type of nutrition problem	Situation	Appropriate nutritional surveillance system
A. Chronic	Government policies/programmes that affect nutrition, that are open to modification on nutritional grounds, and/or that have nutritional objectives **or** Large-scale food distribution and health programmes **or** Need to identify and intention to initiate new programmes aimed at nutrition, basic needs, etc.	Nutritional surveillance for health and development planning
B. Chronic and/or acute	Programmes whose objectives include improvement in nutrition/basic needs **and** Management organization that can adjust the programme on the basis of regular evaluations of outcome	Evaluation of adequacy of programmes using nutritional surveillance methods
C. Acute	Rapid fluctuations in food availability at household level (e.g., due to drought, seasonal factors) **and** Resources and organization for interventions to prevent these fluctuations and/or their effects **and** Lack of adequate information to trigger and target these interventions (acting as a constraint)	Timely warning and intervention programme

the users of the information to be produced, (c) the feasibility and cost of obtaining and analysing the required data. Table 2.1 shows possible combinations of circumstances that will determine the objectives of nutritional surveillance. These are discussed briefly here; the steps described in the rest of this chapter relate to this framework.

Support for health and development planning, usually at national level, is the first objective of nutritional surveillance under the conditions shown in Table 2.1 (A). Government policies and programmes – in a number of sectors – have a substantial effect on nutrition, even if this is not their main objective. One approach to improving nutrition in the long term involves assessing these effects and seeking to enhance them. This procedure requires information, and nutritional surveillance may be a suitable means of obtaining this. When nutrition units are established in the central government with the objective of orienting government activities towards improving nutrition, setting up a nutritional surveillance system for this purpose is generally part of their activities; this has been the case, for example, in Kenya and Sri Lanka. Similarly, health ministries in several countries are building up nutritional information systems. Large-scale food distribution and health programmes require information for planning, and eventually for evaluation. Here, the needs for nutritional surveillance are in principle clearer; moreover, the programmes themselves can provide the required resources for surveillance. Such programmes in several countries in Latin America (e.g., Colombia, Costa Rica) include nutritional surveillance systems. Evidently these are also likely to serve the needs of programme evaluation.

The design of nutritional surveillance for programme management and evaluation differs from that of surveillance for planning purposes, in terms of organization, data needs, sampling procedures, and so on. This is why this objective needs to be distinguished from the outset. These differences arise because the system is closely linked to one particular programme, usually being carried out in one area of a country rather than at national level. As shown in Table 2.1 (B), such programmes may be aimed at acute or chronic problems of malnutrition. It is worth considering setting up nutritional surveillance in relation to such programmes when nutritional improvement is an explicit objective; and when the management of the programme is in a position to respond to information about the programme and its effects during programme implementation.

Timely warning and intervention programmes are needed in closely defined circumstances, as shown in Table 2.1 (C). Intermittent food shortages cause acute malnutrition in many countries: these are frequently seasonal, but may also be less predictable, resulting from drought, changes in economic conditions, and so on. Even if an occurrence of food shortage is not sufficiently severe to be regarded as famine it may still cause widespread suffering and contribute extensively to the overall problem of malnutrition in a country. This is so in many places where seasonal shortages are experienced, in regions as diverse as Indonesia and East Africa. Often in these circumstances a procedure already exists to deal with the effects of, at least, unusual food shortages. If such problems have a priority claim on resources, it can be decided to build up a timely warning and intervention programme combining a predetermined set of interventions with the minimum information needed to initiate these in time to prevent the effects of food shortage. This is covered here as a third possible type of nutritional surveillance – with characteristics in terms of data, analyses, and organization that are quite distinct from those of the other types.

The steps in the initial assessment, illustrated in Table 2.2, are now discussed in more detail.

Table 2.2. Steps in initial assessment for designing a nutritional surveillance system

Purposes of step [a]	Actions to be taken
A. Identification of users, decisions to be taken, and hence purposes and types of surveillance required	Draw up lists of: — policies and programmes currently or potentially impinging on (a) those most affected by nutritional problems and (b) the causes of these problems — ministries, departments, and institutions responsible for potentially relevant actions (planning, implementation, evaluation) Hence define: — existing policies and programmes relevant to nutrition — institutions that are possible users of nutritional surveillance information — decisions to be taken now or in the future that require information, and existing information basis — information needed by relevant institutions for planning, initiation of programmes, monitoring and evaluation
B. Identification of problems	Decide on: — type of malnutrition and whether chronic or acute — groups affected, in geographical and socioeconomic terms — causes of malnutrition in these groups
C. Specification of information needed and baseline statement	Draw up summary statement of what is currently known about nutritional problems: — use actual figures, presented as tables, maps, graphs, etc. — hence identify gaps in information needed for decision-making Identify sources of data from those already used in initial assessment, plus e.g., — data routinely available, if at present not used, from administrative sources — possibility of including nutrition variables in household surveys Assess the suitability of the data for surveillance purposes — variables, level of aggregation, linkage with other data, regularity, timing, reliability, etc.
D. Institutional arrangements	Decide on: — organizational and analysis unit, including staffing — linkages to decision-making — means of supporting field operations, including need to hire staff for data collection and supervision

[a] These steps are iterative, not sequential.

Identifying Users and Decisions (see Table 2.2A)

The purpose of this stage is to specify as clearly as possible the decisions and actions that are being, or could be, taken to improve nutrition. This assessment, together with the information culled from the existing data sources should lead to a preliminary decision on which way to go. The decisions involved concern:

- the institutions that use the surveillance outputs;
- the activities that need to be initiated and supported;
- the administrative level involved (e.g., national or local government);
- and hence the major objective of the surveillance activities.

Usually this process requires investigation by those designing the surveillance system, and it is most important that this be done in close consultation with all concerned. No general prescription is possible. Identifying users and potential decisions is specific to any situation, may be highly political, and requires discussion and negotiation. It also depends on where the initiative to set up a nutritional surveillance system originates – who in effect is carrying out the initial assessment. This may be done by potential users, data producers, or both. The steps given here have not all been carried out systematically in the design of any one system, but experience shows that they should all be brought in when the system is being considered. They are not sequential but iterative. They are outlined in Table 2.2 (A).

One early step is to identify the policies and programmes that in practice are affecting nutrition and discuss them with the government ministries and agencies responsible. In the first instance, this approach should be comprehensive; it will quickly become clear on further enquiry which ministries or agencies are likely to utilize nutritional information for decision-making. Such an inventory could be drawn up along the lines of the following examples:

- environment ministry: subsidized distribution of basic foods;
- agricultural ministry: commodity production programmes;
- rural development agency: area development programmes;
- health ministry: distribution of environmental and primary health care services;
- economic planning ministry: overall budgetary allocations by sector and area;
- national marketing board: producer and consumer food prices;
- local government: public works programmes.

At the level of national planning, the relevant decisions may involve regional allocation of resources, agricultural and food policies (self-sufficiency, pricing, production pattern, marketing), distribution of health and social welfare services, etc. At lower administrative levels (province, state, etc.) further decisions on allocation of resources, on programme design, and on needs for evaluation may be appropriate. The relevance of these decisions to nutritional problems, the possibility of influencing the decisions, and the requirement for new programmes, lead to a preliminary identification of the users of nutritional surveillance information. In other circumstances – again depending upon where the initiative comes from – the primary user of the system may be clear from the outset. This is the case when a well-established programme is supporting the surveillance programme. Even then, however, consideration of other potential users can lend further justification to the surveillance programme.

The next step is to select those user institutions, and the relevant decisions, that will be supported as a matter of priority. The problems, and associated causes, to be tackled (see next section) need to be considered in making this selection. At the same time, the data available must be interpreted to provide a basis for decision-making by the institutions potentially involved – this is also discussed in the next section. This amounts to a pretesting of the usefulness of possible outputs of a surveillance system; if there is a genuine need for information, the initial assessment begins to meet this need and thus ensures that the need is real and more closely specifies the ways in which it can best be met. For example, in Costa Rica much of the first two years of the nutrition information system's activities were taken up with an analysis of existing data; this led to an increase in the potential users beyond the immediate programme supporting the surveillance system and to the information serving a broader range of users. In the Philippines, as a second example, production of sample outputs led to the identification of potential users of nutritional information prepared to support programmes ranging from food distribution to integrated rural development.

During this process, the issues concerning current (or future) policies and programmes, on which decisions affecting nutrition are made, must be understood. The costs and benefits involved in being better able to include nutrition objectives in these programmes must be considered. Hence the real difference that better nutritional data may make must be assessed.

The gaps in existing nutritional information, which a surveillance system could fill, can thus be identified. On occasions, this may be a matter of insufficient sample size to allow an adequately disaggregated analysis of the problems: this has been the case in Kenya, for example, and is being rectified with an expanded sample. Alternatively, reliability of data may be a problem. In general, factors of concern include coverage (e.g., sample surveys give a wide range of variables, but census results may be needed for accurate targeting); availability of data over time to assess deterioration and improvement; addition of descriptive variables to assess causal factors and hence the relevance of different programmes; and other factors, discussed in Chapter 4.

These decisions increasingly depend on an assessment of the priority problems to be tackled – considerations that guide the process and give a basis for discussion. How priority problems can be determined is now outlined. Based on this, more details of assessing data needs are then put forward.

Deciding Which Problems to Tackle

Bringing together knowledge of the types of nutritional deficiency, their magnitude and geographical distribution, periodicity of occurrence, and underlying socioeconomic factors is a part of the initial assessment (see Table 2.2 B). For example, if a country has never experienced famines, and if this is clearly noted in the initial assessment, timely warning and intervention would not be a major purpose of the surveillance system. On the other hand, if the extent of malnutrition varies by region or by socioeconomic group, the appropriate system may be one whose major purpose is to support health and development planning efforts. As a third case, it may be important to ascertain the nutritional effects and administrative aspects of current programmes. Then a major purpose of the system may be evaluation of such programmes. Thus, identification of nutritional deficiencies and socioeconomic problems will modify preconceptions about the main purposes of nutritional surveillance.

A basic statement is needed describing approximately the extent of malnutrition, which deficiencies are important, and the nature and size of the groups affected. This way of describing nutritional problems is illustrated in Fig. 2.1. Such a statement provides the necessary background for deciding on uses, decisions, and data needs. Moreover, it is changes in indicators of these nutritional problems that nutritional surveillance will be designed to follow or predict.

Fig. 2.1. Ways of describing problems

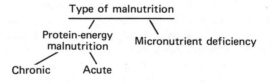

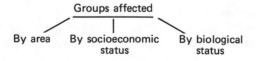

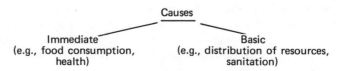

WHO 83643

Malnutrition does not affect everyone in a society to the same extent or for the same reasons. The most common type of nutritional problem is protein–energy malnutrition (PEM). Micronutrient deficiencies – usually of vitamin A, iron, or iodine – may affect population groups different from those suffering from PEM. Protein–energy malnutrition is usually the predominant form, and is the main concern of the nutritional surveillance considered here. The existence and prevalence of protein–energy malnutrition, and of micronutrient deficiencies, is documented, at least roughly, in almost all countries. Accurate data on overall prevalences are not needed, at least at this stage. Some consideration of the severity of malnutrition is required, including its relation to infant and child mortality rates. The indicators for the initial assessment are the same, in principle, as the outcome indicators for nutritional surveillance, as discussed in detail in later chapters.

For planning a surveillance system, it is more important to examine who is affected than to strive for accurate overall measures of malnutrition. This question needs to be tackled partly in relation to possible actions, by using both area and socioeconomic classifications of the population affected by malnutrition. This classification is also needed to assess the appropriateness of present or future actions. Certain programmes are targeted by area, for example health services. Others, particularly those affecting resource and income distribution, are in practice targeted by other criteria, such as occupation or resource endowment. The definition of individual biological status is perhaps the least useful for two reasons. First, because the most biologically vulnerable groups (e.g., infants and preschool children) are much the same everywhere; secondly, because many policies and programmes can only be targeted at household groups and not at individuals within the household. The early outputs from many nutritional surveillance systems have provided information of this type – giving indicators of nutritional conditions by geographical and socioeconomic groupings – and a number of examples are given later. Such indicators have not usually been regarded as part of an initial assessment since most systems have not gone through this phase. How this step is regarded is not important; what matters is to produce such results, from existing data, at an early stage in order to promote discussion and to decide which problems should be given priority.

Causes can be assessed to different degrees, and this assessment must be related to specific problems, groups affected, and hence to possible remedial measures. This question has been discussed in Chapter 1, pp. 18-20, where the potential causes of malnutrition, ranging from resource distribution to weaning practices, are examined. The main objectives at this initial assessment stage are, firstly, to ensure that there is some shared understanding of the causes of malnutrition among those concerned with design of the surveillance system; and secondly to delineate the extent to which basic causes can be tackled with government policies and programmes. For example, almost always malnutrition is closely associated with poverty; the causes of malnutrition are therefore, at one level, the same as the causes of poverty. Inadequate purchasing power for food and a hostile sanitary environment are results – or part of – poverty and are more specific causes of malnutrition. In some circumstances, nutritional information may be used to influence resource allocations for tackling poverty in general, for example as integrated development programmes or policies affecting resource distribution. In this case, nutrition will only be one of many factors considered (no government is going to change important policies on the basis of nutrition alone). More often, nutrition information (including assessment of causes) may be used for identifying and addressing specific factors (which are, of course, aspects of poverty) related to malnutrition: water supplies or food prices, for example. Since the assessment of causes can be virtually open-ended, this procedure can be brought within useful bounds only by relating it systematically to actions that it is realistic to consider the government might undertake, at least partly, for nutritional reasons. Being realistic does not mean being faint-hearted. Where there is need for far-reaching changes these should be discussed. This process includes, therefore, a sounding out of the potential users of nutritional surveillance as to which decisions are likely to be based, even if only to a limited extent, on nutrition. Having done this, some finalization must be reached as to which institutions and decisions require information, to the extent that they will have a genuine effect on the causes of malnutrition problems.

These three questions – types of problem, who is affected, and causes – may be addressed using the same basic data along with local knowledge and common sense. This part of the initial assessment need not be very elaborate, but it needs to be done. The analysis of data identifies nutritional problems, lends credibility to any statements made, and produces figures that potential users can react to. The analytical procedures involve disaggregating the available data so that they refer to easily identifiable groups of the population affected.

Problem identification should not claim a major proportion of the resources available for initial assessment. The effort needed depends partly on the magnitude of the problem and on the need to gain political support, but must not serve as an excuse for avoiding doing something concrete about malnutrition. On the other hand, it is not always widely understood what the problem and its causes really are, and hence what needs to be done and for whom. Preconceived notions of required actions have frequently turned out to be wrong in the past.

What Information is Needed – Outputs and Data Sources

Deciding on what information should be produced by the surveillance system for purposes that are now at least preliminarily identified needs a balance between feasibility, with existing resources, and usefulness. Figures concentrate the mind. In the initial assessment, example outputs should be produced from existing data, even if this requires time and resources; if there simply are no useful data, which is unlikely but possible, this may show that another preliminary step is required involving initial data collection and analysis. Some of these data will have been needed for consideration of which problems to tackle. However, it may be necessary to go beyond this to produce example outputs which would fill information gaps, and to draw up dummy tables of other outputs that may be required. Certain devices, such as mapping, may increase the impact of the presentation.

The hypothetical outputs have to be matched to the objectives of the system being designed. Planning at national level will usually require some information covering the country as a whole, but it may well be decided to concentrate resources on certain areas or groups identified in the initial assessment as being particularly affected by malnutrition or at high risk. The required periodicity of data collection may be every one or two years, as opposed to more frequent outputs needed for other purposes. Where programme evaluation is a priority, some analysis of what is known about the effectiveness of certain existing programmes may be in order. Often this turns out to be not very much. Programme administrators often want to have a system that gives net outcome (or impact) and to have this done internally rather than be subject to outside evaluations. Surveillance, as pointed out in Chapter 5, can deliver adequacy evaluation (i.e., monitoring of gross outcome not impact), as part of programme management. This compromise may or may not be acceptable but it must be noted. In focusing on acute food shortages for timely warning and intervention, a historical view of these events may be helpful in showing how these might have been predicted, and where the necessary information might come from in the future.

Although it will, to some extent, already have been taken care of in earlier steps, exploring possible sources of data should be included in this late stage of the initial assessment. This exploration usually leads back to reconsidering the feasibility of emerging designs for surveillance systems. Very often suitable data collection mechanisms exist, and the trick is to use data already being collected and, where necessary, to introduce nutrition measurements into these.

The suitability of different data sources again depends on the purpose of the surveillance system. This is illustrated in Table 2.3. Some of the most useful sources are introduced below, and more details are given in Chapters 4–6.

Several sources of routine administrative data are in use at present in surveillance systems (see Chapter 4). Most commonly data are obtained from the health system; for example, anthropometric and morbidity data are obtained from clinics. Heights and weights of schoolchildren are often available from schools, although these sources are not yet very widely used. Agricultural and health reporting systems are not uncommon, and can provide excellent opportunities for building up nutritional surveillance systems. Multipurpose household surveys are common in many developing countries. There is thus a possibility of including a nutrition module in these to give data relevant to nutrition. In addition, single-purpose surveys, such as those concerned with the household budget, fertility, or the labour force, can be used to derive relevant

Table 2.3. Suitability of different data sources
for nutritional surveillance purposes

Purpose of surveillance	Suitable data sources
Health and development planning	Household surveys, using data already collected and including nutrition measurements Nutrition and related data collected by government services: health statistics, education data, administrative records (including birth and death registration), agricultural reporting, census statistics
Programme management and evaluation	Inclusion of nutrition measurements in monitoring and evaluation systems Data obtained from programme contacts by interviews and measurements Programme records Intermittent small-scale surveys
Timely warning and intervention programmes	Data on rainfall, prices, employment, and other variables on which routine reports are made Nutrition information collected through existing sources, e.g., the health system Ad hoc surveys

indicators. Programme monitoring and evaluation systems are in operation for many large-scale development programmes, again providing opportunities for setting up nutritional surveillance for evaluation purposes; more details are given in Chapter 5.

The net for data sources should be cast wide at the beginning. There is a trade-off between newness of data, rate of expected change, and timing of decisions; hence, certain data, even several years old, may still be useful. At the same time, such factors as volume of data available, ability to handle this, and needs for identified decisions must be assessed. The degree of aggregation of the available data, the possibility of linking them with other variables, their regularity, and their periodicity of reporting will all need to be considered. Constraints associated with undefined coverage of many administrative data need to be realistically assessed as well. None the less, a principle of surveillance is to use whatever usable data are at hand. In very poor countries with widespread problems of malnutrition and minimal development of statistical services, the only option may be to use whatever data are available from administrative services. In countries higher up the income scale, which tend to have better developed institutional capacity as regards data collection and analysis, sample survey methods may be included. Where administrative capacity is more developed still and government services have wider coverage, generally in more developed countries, more reliance may be put on data derived from routine services, supported by survey work.

Institutional Arrangements and Resource Requirements

The organization of a nutritional surveillance system is going to be to some extent intersectoral under most circumstances. This may be at the level of data collection, analysis, data use, or all of these. The prerequisites are, first, the authority and mandate to collect certain types of data; secondly, the resources to collect, analyse, and interpret the data; and thirdly, linkages to relate results to decision-making. Details of existing institutional arrangements, which may act as some guide, are given in Chapters 3 and 4.

For systems aimed at planning, the main institutional focus is a central unit or group responsible for collating, analysing, and interpreting data, and presenting results and recommendations to other government departments. The units themselves do not always have responsibility for the actual data collection, and not directly for the decisions made based on the information outputs. For programme evaluation, the main focus is within the programme being monitored and evaluated; in effect, responsibility lies with the programme's management, although additional expertise is periodically required for design, some aspects of analysis, etc. In a timely warning and intervention programme, the system should ideally be run or supervised by those with authority to launch the interventions necessary to prevent deterioration; this is not always the case, which is one of the constraints on the effectiveness of these systems.

Along with decisions about who uses a system, information requirements, and data sources, the initial assessment will, most importantly, have to lead to conclusions on institutional arrangements and organization of the surveillance system. Almost the first decision will be whether the focus should be at national or area level. This depends primarily on where the decision-making power lies. But the existence of the necessary organization and analytical capability is also crucial, and this is less often available at local than at national level. If local surveillance programmes are decided upon it is likely that training from a central unit, and periodic assistance, may be needed.

Organization for data collection, whether from administrative sources or surveys, will depend partly on using the time of people already employed for purposes other than nutritional surveillance. A hard-headed look at what can reasonably be expected of these staff is needed. Often the data collection agencies will already exist, the ''surveillance unit'' being attached to a planning body; in this case, a clear understanding as to responsibility for data collection is needed. Decisions will also be needed on whether to employ further staff for supervision and possibly data gathering. For example, employment of staff to visit schools, clinics, local registrars, etc., might well ensure a reliable flow of data – often with record sampling at the source – and provide some check on the reliability of the data themselves. Similarly, additional staff to train enumerators in a sample survey system, and perhaps to provide some supervision, may be needed. Whether these staff will be supported by, and be responsible to, the data collection agency or the central unit will need to be decided.

Data analysis, particularly in systems whose main purpose is to support planning, will often need to be centralized, usually at national level, although larger countries may have the capacity at one or more administrative levels. Here, adequate resources of skilled personnel will be a constraint. Nutrition institutions may help – but careful links must be set up to avoid problems when these institutions are not closely related to points of decision. A distinction may also be needed between routine uncomplicated analysis, which may be usefully decentralized, and more sophisticated analyses requiring expertise that is not widely available.

It is usually necessary to set up a central unit for each surveillance programme, and making resources available for this constitutes one of the crucial decisions in setting up a system. The institution responsible will often be the same as that undertaking the initial assessment. This unit itself may be within a larger institution and draw on the resources of this, for example, within a statistical office. Looking at present surveillance systems it is clear that several full-time staff are needed in order to establish anything worth while. Certain of these full-time staff need professional skills and access to others on a part-time basis will also be required. The skills needed are in subjects such as nutrition, statistics, economics, agriculture, health, and (often) computer science – depending on the type and focus of the system.

The institutional needs for linking information to decision-making are likely to include some form of intersectoral coordinating body. The central unit acts partly as the secretariat to this body. This must have representation at a sufficiently high level to be able to influence policy, and often to have access to plans at an early stage. For this purpose, it may be possible to build on to an existing arrangement for dealing with nutritional matters within the government.

Procedures for disseminating information need to be considered, although these can develop with the system. A combination of informal reports – through meetings, professional contacts, etc. – regular summary bulletins, and periodic in-depth publications is likely to be suitable. Regular communication between users, at all levels, must be designed into the programme, not only to communicate information from the system, but also to review the ways in which this information is itself disseminated.

Work-plan for a Surveillance System

Finally, all these considerations must be brought together as a practical work-plan for building up a surveillance system. In the case of a review of an ongoing programme, this work-plan serves a similar function, updating the existing plan. The work-plan should detail who does what (the responsibilities assigned to different cooperating agencies), the budget, and a schedule of activities and outputs.

In summary, at the end of the initial assessment, those promoting and/or responsible for nutritional surveillance will have a clear view of the types of nutritional deficiences and problems they are tackling, the political feasibility, and the support likely to be available (in terms of the necessary institutional arrangements and human and economic resources allocated to surveillance), and other actions aimed at improving nutrition. At the same time, the effort will also illustrate the technical problems that will arise in setting up the information system and thus the number of personnel and their qualifications. Finally, the initial identification of users and uses, the mechanisms for dissemination of the information, and the type and periodicity of data outputs will be of utmost importance in designing a nutritional surveillance system to meet the selected purposes.

REFERENCES

1. WHO Technical Report Series, No. 593, 1976 (*Methodology of nutritional surveillance. Report of a Joint FAO/UNICEF/WHO Expert Committee*).

CHAPTER 3

Nutritional surveillance for health and development planning: uses and organization

Summary

Nutritional surveillance makes possible better-informed decisions on ways of preventing or alleviating malnutrition. These decisions concern adjustments in current policies and programmes, initiation of new measures, and targeting of both health/ nutrition and development programmes. The information needed for these decisions concerns: relative nutritional conditions in different population groups and characteristics associated with malnutrition; how the nutrition situation is changing, overall and for different groups, and characteristics associated with the changes; and identification of specific problems or trends towards these. Broadly speaking, this information is used within national development plans for targeting large-scale programmes and for identifying smaller-scale measures for specific problems. Such information has been used in national plans in several countries with surveillance systems (e.g., Costa Rica, Kenya, Philippines); and for targeting health and food distribution programmes, for example, in Colombia and Costa Rica.

The organization of nutritional surveillance, focused on surveillance units, involves ensuring the function of components of the system – data collection, data analysis, and inputs to decision-making – and of linkages between these components, that is, a flow of data from collection to interpretation. Several sectors of government are usually concerned, as regards both collection and use of the data. An insufficiency of data is seldom the problem; common problems concern sampling of data (often of records collected) and feed-back. Data handling involves management of analysis by computer, often requiring cooperation with several institutions outside the surveillance system itself. Some lessons can be drawn from analogous information systems: health information systems, agricultural reporting systems, and household sample surveys. Existing institutions, including nutrition institutions and those already concerned with information (government statistical offices and data units within ministries of health and agriculture, for example) have an important role to play. The manpower resources required to establish nutritional surveillance depend on how far these cooperating institutions are able to cooperate, but experience shows that a minimum of about five full-time professional staff are usually needed to form a surveillance unit: this is similar to the requirements for other data units.

Background

This chapter describes nutritional surveillance systems that provide information useful for health and development planning and discusses the ways in which such information can be used for decision-making. The data needs are covered in Chapter 4. The aim of these two chapters is twofold. First, they offer guidance in deciding whether and how to set up nutritional surveillance programmes in support of decisions on how to improve nutrition. Secondly, they provide information of more general interest to those concerned with nutrition on the ways in which decisions are taken, on how information is obtained, and on what it means.

Reviews of progress in nutritional surveillance were initiated in 1979 by both the Sub-Committee on Nutrition of the Administrative Committee on Coordination (ACC-SCN) and the National Academy of Sciences of the USA. In 1980, this work was continued by the Cornell Nutritional Surveillance Program. The results were presented at an International Workshop on Nutritional Surveillance, held in Cali, Colombia, in July 1981. The reviews begun in 1979 elicited information from some 18 nutritional surveillance programmes in different parts of the world. Much of what follows is based upon the 18 programmes studied, as well as on experience in related information systems – health information systems, agricultural reporting systems, and household surveys. Other programmes not included, or not selected as particular examples in the text, are in no way considered less important; it is merely that we know much less about them.

The order in which nutritional surveillance systems are described is the reverse of that usually followed – and indeed the reverse of the chronology of their operation. This is because, as for the initial assessment described in Chapter 2, it is necessary to start by deciding what one is trying to achieve, and then how to do it, and not the other way around. For this reason this chapter first describes the uses of nutritional surveillance for decision-making, and then how to obtain the necessary information, including examples of how certain existing systems work.

Objectives and Questions to be Answered

The overall objective of nutritional surveillance is to promote actions that will alleviate or prevent malnutrition by providing better information on which to base planning decisions with respect to nutrition. In principle, these decisions include:

(a) whether to modify current or planned policies and programmes in the light of the existing nutrition situation, changes in this, and its causes;

(b) whether to initiate new measures to improve nutrition, and for whom;

(c) how to target programmes in order to have the desired effect on nutrition.

Certain types of information must be produced to facilitate these decisions. But even more important, this information must be made available in an institutional setting that ensures as far as possible that it is acted upon: establishing and fostering a mechanism for decision-making is itself an important objective of nutritional surveillance.

A useful way of defining the information required is by preparing a set of questions. In order to be useful for health and development planning, a nutritional surveillance system should be designed to provide answers to the

Table 3.1. Questions that need to be answered
by nutritional surveillance information to aid health
and development planning decisions

	Question	Output	Planning implication
1. (a)	Are there certain areas/ people with appreciably worse nutritional conditions than others, and what are their characteristics?	Initial assessment; one-time disaggregated data by region and socioeconomic status	Targeting of interventions; assessment of causes and hence of relevance of existing policies and programmes; preliminary assessment of size of problems, hence of initial resource implications
(b)	Which characteristics are most closely associated with the outcome? [a]		
2. (a)	Is the overall health, nutrition, and socioeconomic situation deteriorating or improving?	Aggregated data, over time	General view of situation; if general improvement, need to look at rate and at specific groups; if general deterioration, need for concern for overall position, as well as for groups
(b)	Is the trend the same for all groups, or are there some groups showing a different trend?	Disaggregated data, over time	Targeting. Reassessment of problems; identification of intervention measures; resource allocations and procuring additional resources
(c)	How are deteriorating or lagging groups defined?	Disaggregated data, over time, with classifications	
(d)	What characteristics are associated with differences in trend? [a]	Disaggregated data, over time, with classifications	More specific identification of causes of change, hence interventions and policy changes needed
3. (a)	Is a specific short-term problem indicated (e.g., food shortage, epidemic)?	Only one (or a few) outcome indicator(s) sharply deteriorating	Specific interventions needed
(b)	Are there fluctuations that indicate recurrent short-term deterioration?	Disaggregated data, over time	Preventive measures
(c)	Are there trends that indicate probable crisis in the future?	Disaggregated data, over time	Preventive measures

[a] Dependent variable is, for question 1, outcome; for question 2, change in outcome.

questions in Table 3.1. The table shows the data outputs required to answer these questions (middle column). Individual questions do not necessarily refer to only one of the decisions (*a*) to (*c*) outlined above; rather, each question can give additional information relevant to all of these. These questions provide the theme running through much of this chapter and are now discussed in more detail.

Questions 1 (*a*) and 1 (*b*) in Table 3.1 can be answered from cross-sectional data (obtained on one occasion). Determining whether there are areas or population groups with particular problems begins in the initial assessment (Chapter 2) and involves disaggregating data by suitable descriptive variables. The relative importance of descriptive factors in distinguishing the prevalence of malnutrition by group may be investigated by more advanced statistical analyses. These outputs are relevant both to targeting and to obtaining insights into causal factors. They thus provide information for assessing existing programmes and the need for further measures.

Surveillance is clearly distinguished from surveys and one-time assessments by the second set of questions (2(*a*) to 2(*d*) in Table 3.1). Assessing changes over time greatly increases the usefulness of the results. In practice, the first issue generally refers to the overall situation – is it getting better or worse? Using this information requires knowledge of whether everyone is changing at the same rate, or whether the average changes are accounted for mainly by changes in certain sections of the population (question 2(*b*)). Obviously, if the trends for certain groups of people show sharp deteriorations, the need for further measures is clearly indicated. The reasons for such changes may be obvious or may need further investigation. Again, some clues will be available from the characteristics of the groups showing change (question 2(*c*)), and further studies of the association of these characteristics with changes in outcome indicators may be needed (question 2(*d*)). A particular reason for investigating changes in relation to their causes is for the purposes of programme management and evaluation, which are subjects dealt with in Chapter 5: question 2(*d*) provides the link with evaluation.

The third set of questions brings to light specific problems of either current or possible future importance. The answers may show the need for more immediate action, for example, to prevent the effects of a developing food shortage or of decreasing purchasing power (question 3(*a*)). Beyond this, a longer-term programme, including provisions for timely warning and intervention (see Chapter 6) may be required (question 3(*b*)). Finally, when more extensive time-series data are available, underlying trends may be observed that give warning of problems in the future that are not yet so urgent, but for which preventive measures should now be considered to reverse the trend (question 3(*c*)).

Uses of Information for Decisions

Determining the ways in which data have been used for decision-making in practice presents certain problems. First, the processes of decision-making are sometimes not based on published material, but on informal communications. Secondly, the process is often not documented and the decisions themselves are not always published. Documented examples of surveillance data being used for planning are therefore infrequent at present. In part, this may reflect extensive under-utilization of data, because either the institutional links are weak, or the data are presented so that the policy implications are not made explicit. Perhaps, also, it is too early in the development of surveillance systems to expect such examples to be widely available. None the less, the recorded uses can be summarized as follows:

— for national development plans and policy directives;
— for targeting large-scale national social welfare, food, and nutrition programmes;
— for identifying specific problems requiring special attention.

These uses relate directly to the different ways in which nutrition problems can be tackled, as described on p. 29-37. Thus nutritional information has been used in policy-making in relation to national development plans, and in selecting certain programmes for priority attention. The use of nutritional data for targeting is observed mainly where there are large national programmes that require such data. Such uses are best illustrated by examples, as described below.

Development plans and policy directives

In Costa Rica, the general awareness of nutrition has been enhanced by the activities of the *Sistema de Información en Nutrición* (SIN) (*1*). The Family Allowances Programme supports the SIN, and is the main user of the information produced. The activities of the Family Allowances Programme are assessed for their relevance, cost, and coverage using SIN data. The SIN data are also used centrally by the global planning division of the planning office. This unit in the Ministry of Planning has developed a basic-needs strategy drawing substantially on the nutritional data. A third example of the use of the SIN data is in reviewing export policies for rice (the main staple), which are adjusted on the basis of estimated trends in food-energy and protein available from basic grains. In fact, the data are being used more and more as their availability becomes better known throughout the Government.

In Kenya, nutritional data were collected as past of the Integrated Rural Surveys. These data and the results of the agro-economic and environmental components of the Surveys were used in the 1979-83 National Development Plan. This plan included a summary of nutritional problems in relation to economic factors based substantially on the nutritional data. The Government wished to strengthen the plan's focus on nutrition and basic needs and as a first step a food and nutrition planning unit was established in the planning ministry. This unit had a mandate to coordinate activities in the different sectors, to review policies and programmes as regards their nutritional impact, and to focus them on particular nutritional problems. The unit operates through an interministerial coordinating committee on nutrition and draws on the nutritional information from the Central Bureau of Statistics.

In the Philippines, the results of the nation-wide community weighing programme have been used in annual and five-year plans (1978–82) for the Philippine Nutrition Program (2). Information on the extent of preschool malnutrition and its distribution between administrative areas has contributed to some allocation of resources to the nutrition programmes in depressed regions. These data have also been used by the National Economic Development Authority to help identify priority areas. A number of policy directives in support of the nutrition programme have been based on these results.

The Food and Nutrition Policy Planning Division in Sri Lanka has access to nutritional information from many sources. These include the 1976 survey that was assisted by the Centers for Disease Control (USA), the pilot nutritional surveillance project under the Medical Research Institute (Colombo), and numerous other surveys. Data from these sources have been used for policy decisions, evaluation, and modification of feeding programmes.

Targeting and control of national programmes

Decisions have been mainly on targeting by administrative area. In Colombia, the *Plan de Alimentación y Nutrición* (PAN) is at present targeted in this way, on the basis of data from the two-yearly surveys carried out under the PAN's auspices. State governments are setting up surveillance systems, based on a pilot model developed by the Universidad del Valle, Cali, which are to provide for more precise targeting in the future. In Costa Rica, the SIN data have led to a number of targeting decisions. The best-known example refers to eleven cantons which were identified by means of nutritional and other indicators as worst-affected. These cantons were declared by presidential decree as being of priority, and additional resources from the Family Allowances Programme were assigned to them. In the Philippines targeting is based on estimated prevalences of malnutrition both at local and at central government levels.

The use of nutritional surveillance data for evaluation and management of programmes is discussed further in Chapter 5.

Identification of specific problems

Information from nutritional surveillance sometimes highlights new or poorly understood problems. The prevalence of malnutrition, or of other health status indicators such as child mortality, may be particularly high for one group or area. Alternatively, nutritional status may be out of line with other indicators, for instance those reflecting wealth or access to services. In such cases, special measures would be required to deal with the specific problems. This can be illustrated by two examples.

In Costa Rica, analysis of the 1978 nutrition survey showed that the children of workers in banana plantations had particularly poor nutritional status, although the household income was about average for the country, and other socioeconomic indicators showed nothing unusual.[1] This led to the SIN launching a three-month anthropological study, which identified causes such as contaminated water supply and exceedingly high prices for basic commodities in certain plantations (3, 4). Legislation has been formulated to rectify this situation.

In Sri Lanka, analysis of nutritional data showed that the prevalence of malnutrition (<90% height-for-age) in children of workers on tea estates was about double that for the rest of the country (means of 62% in estates compared with 31% in villages). This was not the only evidence of poor conditions in this group of the population, and the results contributed to a series of measures to improve conditions on the tea estates.

Organization

The purpose of this section is to describe how nutritional surveillance systems work in organizational terms. The components of a system are: data collection; data flow; data processing, analysis and interpretation; and linkage of results to decision-making. Technical details relating to data are given in Chapter 4. Here, the organizational needs are discussed, first, in relation to the way nutritional surveillance and other information systems work at present, and secondly, taking into consideration possible improvements in the future in regard to overall structure, solving particular problems, and use of existing institutions. Finally, some guidance is given concerning resource and staffing requirements.

Existing surveillance systems

Organization of a nutritional surveillance system involves establishing three main components (data collection, data analysis, and inputs to decision-making)

---

[1] Costa Rica. Sistema de Información en Nutrición. *Encuesta nacional de nutrición 1978. Aspectos socioeconómicos de la nutrición*. San José, Oficina de Información, Casa Presidencial, 1980.

and the linkages between them that allow for data flow and transfer of information. A diagram of the way in which these are set up in some existing surveillance systems is given in Fig. 3.1. This figure emphasizes that data are normally drawn from a number of sources within different agencies. All systems have a central unit that is responsible for organization of the system and for data analysis; this may be within a larger organization concerned with data, such as a statistical office, or it may be a unit within a planning or specialized ministry. The outputs of the system go to a number of agencies over and above that to which the central unit is directly attached. The outputs are also used for improving the system itself.

Information systems are focused on an organizing unit. The existing units with responsibility for nutritional surveillance have the following main functions:

— support to sources of data (forms, equipment, training, supervision in some cases);
— organization of data flow;
— analysis and interpretation;
— linkage to planning or programme institutions.

Fig. 3.1. Schematic diagram of surveillance systems
for health and development planning

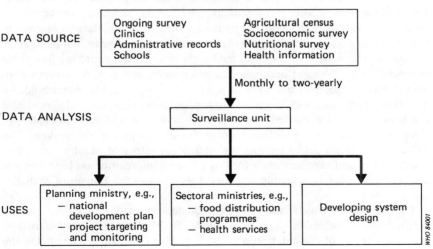

For data obtained from administrative sources, the first responsibility for data collection is with the agencies directly concerned. In the health system, clinics may collect results (for example, weights and ages of children, or presenting illnesses) and transmit these through the usual channels (e.g., district health officer, provincial health officer, etc.) to the analysis unit. Data from schools (for example, heights of schoolchildren) are often summarized by the schoolteacher and again transmitted through normal channels. Other administrative records, such as vital registration, go through local government channels. Census results are, however, normally obtained centrally from the census office.

Most systems rely on computer facilities for handling data. Once received at the central surveillance office, therefore, the data go through conventional procedures for editing and entry to create files for computer processing. The organization at this point requires resources of trained manpower and funds that may not be readily available in some countries.

Up to this point in the procedure, a reasonable amount of experience specific to nutritional surveillance can be drawn on. However, experience in routinely processing and interpreting nutritional data for the purpose of preparing regular reports is limited. The organizational problems at this point have many features in common with other data collection and analysis efforts, such as the operations of government statistical offices or of ministries of health and agriculture. Some of these are considered in a later section.

The organization of collection, flow, and analysis of administrative data in Costa Rica, illustrated in Fig. 3.2, provides an example of many of these mechanisms. The main data sources include the Ministry of Health's rural health and community health programmes, which cover about 60% of the total population. Under these, health workers visit individual families in their homes at least once every 9 weeks. The data made available from these systems are: weights of children from 0 to 6 years old taken every year (approximately 250 000); annual reports on population and family planning, sanitation activities, and vaccinations; annually updated family data; and data on migration, housing conditions, and environmental sanitation every 2 years. Other sources of data include: a national census of the height of all children entering first grade at school every 2 years; occupation, employment, and income surveys conducted every 4 months since 1976 on a national sample of 7000 households by the Ministry of Labor and Social Security; population, housing, and agricultural censuses, which are carried out every 10 years. In addition, in-depth anthropological studies on different occupational groups are undertaken. The Ministry of Health also monitors the nutritional status of children attending health clinics and supplementary feeding centres. Information on birth weights and mortality rates is available annually directly from the Bureau of Statistics and Censuses.

The channels by which data are transmitted depend on the data source. For the height census of schoolchildren, for example, the Ministry of Education used its own mechanism of communication with schools at the village level. On the

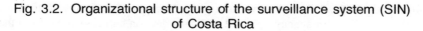

Fig. 3.2. Organizational structure of the surveillance system (SIN) of Costa Rica

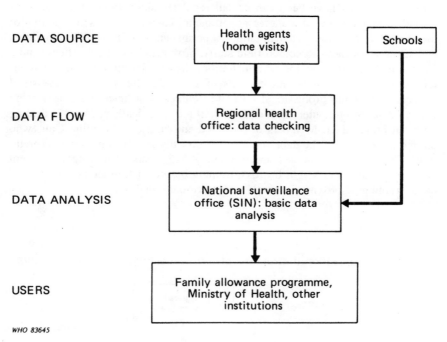

WHO 83645

other hand, health data go up through area health offices. The revision of forms, and the punching, processing, and analyses are conducted centrally by SIN. Computer facilities are available to SIN from the University of Costa Rica and from the Ministry of Finance, the latter facilities being more frequently used. The censuses and the periodic surveys on employment are analysed and reported by the Bureau of Statistics and Censuses and the Ministry of Labor and Social Security, respectively; SIN then incorporates the relevant data into its own reports as needed. The central unit of the SIN employs some 20–30 professionals, with backgrounds in economics, statistics, engineering, data processing, etc.

Data for nutritional surveillance can be derived from sample surveys of households. These data may be obtained by including a nutrition module within a survey system that is already in operation for other purposes; many aspects of the survey organization may thus be taken care of. The inputs for nutritional information involve equipment, training, supervision, data checking, and analysis and interpretation. The organization of these services in Kenya, illustrated in Fig. 3.3, will serve as a good example. The Central Bureau of Statistics is the main agency involved and most data on nutrition come from the rural surveys that have been carried out regularly since 1974. These surveys provide a major source of data for government planning. Successful running of the overall system involves maintaining a permanent field force of enumerators and supervisors (now some 500 field staff), provincial statistical offices, and a central unit responsible for administration, survey design, analysis, and interpretation. This central unit consists of some 20 clerks, several statistical officers, plus senior professional staff and technical assistance. Data processing is carried out by computer. Two or three staff are specifically engaged in dealing with nutritional data. Members of the Food and Nutrition Planning Unit, who are the main users of the data, are also periodically involved in data interpretation. The nutrition modules are run every 2–3 years, requiring equipment (weighing scales and height boards), training before each modular survey (2–3 days' training at provincial level), and nutritional analysis.

Fig. 3.3. Organizational structure of the surveillance system in Kenya

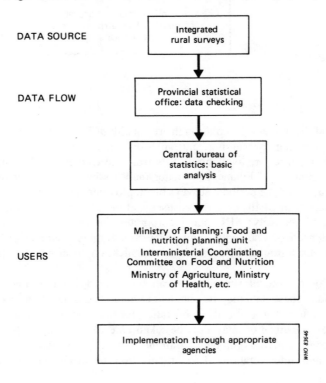

Reporting systems related to nutritional surveillance

Useful experience is available from information systems in related fields, such as health, agriculture and household surveys. These systems are of particular importance since, where they exist or are being developed, they can provide much of the information required for nutritional surveillance. They have the advantage of involving only one sector; while some of the problems of nutritional surveillance may stem from its intersectoral nature, the solutions to others may be suggested by the more extensive experience of health and agricultural systems.

Health information systems

In health information systems, data about a patient's condition are recorded at the time of encounter with the health system – at a clinic or hospital or on a home visit. These records are collated to provide the information necessary for the reports required by the health units. Reports may be sent through a hierarchy of health units or directly to the ministry of health. Analysis may be done at the intermediate level (district or provincial), or by the ministry. Bottlenecks in data flow usually occur because of the time required to summarize and report the information, and because the amount of data to be analysed at the central level is beyond the capacity of the data-handling facilities. Both of these bottlenecks lead to long delays between the time data are collected and information is available for use. The solutions lie in more extensive sampling of records, and greater attention to matching capacity for handling data to the volume of data.

The reporting system in the state of Valle del Cauca, Colombia, is largely based on a health reporting system.[1] Data are obtained on incidence of infectious diseases, mortality from infectious diseases, immunization coverage, birth weight, and anthropometry for any person seen as an outpatient. The data are compiled weekly by assistant statisticians stationed in the health centre, who create a four-weekly listing of new cases, broken down by week and age group. These data are sent every four weeks to the state health department (there are approximately 200 health posts and 40 health centres in the state). While the health information has flowed efficiently, there have been severe problems in handling the volume of nutritional status data collected in the clinics. Approximately 40 000 sets of measurements are available every month, but in the absence of a sampling system it has proved impossible to handle this volume of data. The health data are processed by computer at the university in Cali, and outputs are made available within one month of the data being collected. Reports are sent back to health centres. The other users of the information are at state level, in health, agriculture, education, and social welfare.

[1] Colombia, Fundación para la Educación Superior. *Nutritional Surveillance System. First year progress report, May 15, 1978–May 15, 1979; Second year progress report, May 15, 1979–May 15, 1980.* Cali, Colombia, Nutrition Project, 1979 & 1980 (unpublished documents).

Other, more familiar, disease surveillance systems in developing countries are concerned with rapid reports of notifiable diseases, such as cholera. In these, information is transmitted rapidly, often by cable or telephone, from the clinics that detect outbreaks to the ministry of health. These systems often work well, because there is a clear understanding of the importance at all levels; in addition, and this is most important, there is a predetermined set of actions to combat the problems.

More elaborate disease reporting systems have also been instituted, drawing information from a number of sources, somewhat similar to nutritional surveillance. These are described in the literature on health information systems (5, 6).[1] The potential sources of data in these systems (7) are: birth and death registration, health service statistics, environmental health statistics; accident statistics; etc. Such systems have been tried in several countries, for example, in the United Republic of Cameroon[2] and in the Gambia.[3]

Agricultural reporting systems

Information concerning agriculture may be collected by various agencies in addition to the ministries of agriculture, for example, departments of census and statistics, marketing boards, banks, and agricultural research institutes. Here again, such information could often be used for nutritional surveillance. In ministries of agriculture, data are usually collected from contacts with farmers by extension workers, who send these data on through supervisors to the district office. Some compilation of data may be done along the way. The central ministry then does further analyses and publishes reports. Other sources of data include postal enquiries and surveys by interview. Crop production measurements may be obtained by estimating crop yields on sample areas of crops (crop cutting), combined with estimation of the total crop area. Aerial surveys are occasionally used, but satellite information has not yet been applied in most developing countries. Finally, agricultural censuses (which are in fact sample surveys, rather than a complete enumeration) provide detailed information, but they are infrequent. Certain of these techniques may be combined to give information to forecast crop outputs. These usually involve farmers' reports, sometimes with data from sample surveys. Information is also obtained from marketing boards, but this is mostly for crops when the majority of the output passes through the market.

The difference between running an agricultural reporting system and a health information system is that the data are not collected in the agricultural system unless they are needed at higher administrative levels, whereas many health data

---

[1] See also: *Report of the Interregional Consultation on National Health Information Systems. San José, Costa Rica, 14-20 November 1979.* Geneva, World Health Organization, 1980 (unpublished document).

[2] *Disease surveillance, United Republic of Cameroon.* Atlanta, Centers for Disease Control, 1979.

[3] *Surveillance in Gambia.* Atlanta, Centers for Disease Control, 1980.

are already collected because they are needed for patient treatment. This means that at the level of data collection, there are additional difficulties in maintaining regularity and quality of data in agricultural systems. Further, certain of the measurements, such as crop cutting and area measurements, are particularly difficult to obtain, and the familiar problems of delays in data flow and constraints in data analysis apply to agricultural systems as much as to others. Improving the quality of data has usually involved moving away from reliance on agricultural services themselves and setting up properly organized sample survey systems, with field staff trained for this purpose and closely supervised. Under these conditions, more reliable data are obtained, but generally on a smaller sample than is available through the agricultural services. The handling of such data is more analogous to a household survey system than to a health information system.

Household sample surveys

Household surveys have common features in terms of organization and problems encountered, many of which are independent of whether or not nutrition is included. The organization of household sample surveys is generally well understood and documented (8). Data are obtained by interview, observation and/or measurement. Questionnaire entries are generally checked by a supervisor in the field, and the questionnaires collected together at an area office for further checking, compilation, and transmission to the central office. The data-processing and analytical capacity of the central office is a common constraint. Surveys run by government statistical organizations usually have their own data-handling and analysis arrangements; others, often including those initiated by sectoral ministries, may need to request help with data handling, which can lead to long delays. Moreover, interaction with the data users, who are in yet other institutions, concerning the results of most interest, is not always achieved.

Solving these institutional and organizational problems is central to the successful use of data for both household surveys and nutritional surveillance. As a general rule, it seems that the more the central data analysis unit is in the mainstream of government departments, and the more it has the capacity to analyse and interpret its own data, the more successful it will be in meeting the needs of the users and influencing decision-making. These criteria are thus most often met by statistics units in government departments: central statistical offices within planning ministries and/or serving sectoral ministries; or data units within sectoral ministries themselves. Conversely, research units, commissions, etc., when responsible for data analysis, have more difficulty in making effective use of data for decision-making.

Some organizational issues

The problems of organizing a surveillance system are twofold: (*a*) how to make each component itself function, and (*b*) how to make the links between the components function. These two problems are related and are compounded by the usual need to involve several government agencies. The administrative structure itself may be represented as shown in Fig. 3.4. The compilation, checking, and transmission of the data are often the responsibility of the agency directly concerned until the data reach the central unit. Some analysis may be done at area level, usually for the purposes of the agency involved, e.g., area health programming. Some questions that need attention concerning data collection, flow, handling, and analysis are discussed below.

Data collection and flow

The clinic, school, local government office, etc. will already be collecting certain data in most cases. In others, these resources may be used to obtain additional information. In either case, training, equipment, forms, supervision, and often sampling will be required. These are discussed in Chapter 4. The best way of organizing this data collection is usually through the existing channels of authority, i.e., through the ministry, to the area office, to the village. Supervisors should be trained to train local workers and to supervise data collection; equiment should be channelled through area offices – and training on equipment maintenance given at this level.

Particular issues that are seldom satisfactorily resolved in practice are: sampling, both of data collection sites and of records; and establishing a feedback of information to the collecting point. From a central perspective, the potential volume of data is enormous – increasing logarithmically between each administrative level. At the village level, the last thing a clinic worker or schoolteacher wants is another form to fill out. It has been reported in one instance that at least 400 forms per health centre per year were required. Organization of sampling, of both sites and records, usually needs to be controlled by the central surveillance unit. Often, it is not appreciated that data of satisfactory accuracy can be obtained from a sample. In any event, it is almost always better to obtain some results on a subsample of the available information than to obtain none at all because of failure to analyse a large data set – as has happened on many occasions.

Data flow from village to area office usually involves initial assembling of results at the collecting point, and regular reporting of of these results. Often this is a weaker link than the original data collection. Apart from supervision, one of the ways of maintaining motivation (which is a large part of the problem) is to ensure feedback of results. This question of establishing a two-way flow of information – from those collecting the data to the analytical unit, and subsequent return of the interpretation – has not been satisfactorily resolved. There are two objectives here that need to be separated: first, to feed useful informa-

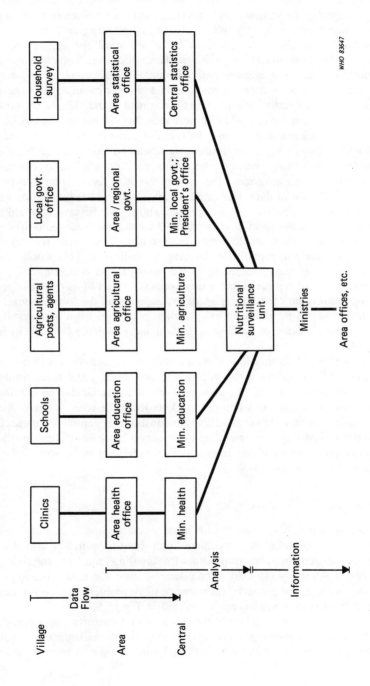

Fig. 3.4. Administrative structure for organization of a nutritional surveillance system

WHO 83647

tion back to the level of data collection to assist in decentralized decision-making; secondly, to motivate and encourage the data collectors to maintain a flow of reliable data. In reality, it is probable that planning authority is seldom sufficiently decentralized for there to be a felt need for aggregated (i.e., "fed-back") information at the point of data collection. Therefore the main issue usually concerns maintaining motivation. This is central to any surveillance system relying on data routinely collected – for example, in clinics. In such cases, data are gathered in relation to treatment of individuals; the problem is not so much one of the reliability of these records as of the satisfactory onward transmission of these results. It may be that this issue has been addressed with insufficient realism, since it is questionable whether a flow of reliable data – in contrast to its collection – will ever be maintained from clinics, for example, if those responsible for preparing the reports are not also responsible for the onward transmission of data. One solution that could be tried would be for the surveillance system itself to employ people whose specific task it would be to extract such data at the point of collection. The exact method would depend on the circumstances: they would either extract data from clinic records or be present periodically to record data as they are collected. This would also be useful in imposing record sampling at the point of data collection.

The extent to which a surveillance unit needs field staff of its own, as opposed to relying entirely on cooperating agencies, depends on the local context. At a minimum, it seems advisable to assign some personnel from the surveillance unit to routine checking of the data collection and to solving bottlenecks in the flow of data.

These bottlenecks in the flow of data usually stem from delays in compiling and checking information at the village and area levels, and transmitting the reports to the next level up. In some cases this is partly tackled by eliminating any intermediate levels, for example, in Costa Rica, the schools report directly to the central ministry. In other cases, the constraint is central – data accumulated in one ministry are not passed on to the surveillance unit. These are clearly managerial problems of prime importance, which need to be solved through interagency agreements.

Data handling and analysis

The organization for data analysis is usually central, and at this level may be more within the control of the surveillance unit. It still requires careful planning and good management. The components for handling data from the field must link together smoothly. Usually a computer is used for data processing, but unless this is organized properly, it can create more problems than it solves. The components of such a system are illustrated in Fig. 3.5.

Making workable arrangements for the regular transformation of raw data from the field into useful reports is no easy task. No surveillance unit at present has a computer section of its own – although the central unit may be part of an

Fig. 3.5. Components of a system for handling data from the field

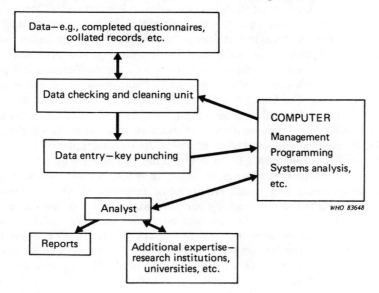

organization that does have its own computer, for example, in a central statistical office. Maintaining a smooth flow between the different parts of the system, therefore, generally requires cooperation between the surveillance unit and other institutions with computer facilities. In addition, expertise in nutrition and other subjects may need to be brought in from specialized bodies, such as universities and research institutions, requiring still further cooperative arrangements.

Another problem is that large volumes of data have proved to be unmanageable. Subsampling of data collected for other purposes (e.g., individual health records) is clearly necessary. Some research on the possible advantages of record sampling, in terms of feasibility of data handling as against accuracy of output, may be needed. Another problem concerns timeliness; the timing of data outputs requires careful definition, and realistic schedules must be agreed upon in advance. Clear definition of the precise outputs needed is essential, and this process should begin in the initial assessment (Chapter 2). Priority should be given to production of time-series data; all too often, data that could be analysed as a time-series are treated cross-sectionally. Considerations such as these should lead to a systematic design of data-handling procedures.

Role of existing institutions

In seeking to develop nutritional surveillance, it is essential that there should be sufficient institutional capacity – mainly people with the necessary skills – to set up and run the system. In fact, many countries have nutrition institutions, or nutrition units within broader structures. The issue is then what priorities should be set for the activities of these institutions. In fact, the fundamental policy question really concerns what can be done to improve nutrition, and what the role of the nutrition institutes in this process should be. As discussed in the first chapter, traditional nutrition programmes may have only limited relevance to tackling problems of malnutrition, and much of what needs to be done lies outside the conventional orbit of nutritionists. An important part of the nutrition institutions' functions could be in contributing to planning by providing the necessary information to other government agencies; in other words, in nutritional surveillance. This would require some switching of existing resources (particularly staff) towards planning and surveillance – and perhaps augmentation of these resources – which in turn might require some retraining and a different emphasis in personnel structure. Such resources do exist in many countries, and a decision could be made to devote part of their capacity to nutritional surveillance. Such a decision would need to be associated with the development of links to other institutions. Nutrition units cannot usually expect to *collect* data themselves; this work will have to be done in collaboration with others: with the agencies on the ground for routine data, and with survey operations for sample survey data. The main roles of the nutrition institutions in surveillance should be concerned with: designing data collection methods, training, assistance in data analysis and interpretation; presentation of results.

Those institutions already concerned with data management in the fields of health, agriculture, economic planning, and statistics are able to contribute much of the expertise necessary for running a nutritional surveillance system. This has been stressed in relation to data collection, but it can also apply to data flow and analysis. Only a small proportion of the people involved in present surveillance systems are professional nutritionists: the majority are, in fact, economists, sociologists, anthropologists, statisticians, agriculturalists, health professionals, etc. People qualified in other disciplines can be trained in quite a short time in most of the aspects of nutrition necessary for working in nutritional surveillance. The less extensive inputs that require a higher level of expertise are then generally available from nutrition institutes in the country concerned, and if necessary from international sources.

Many government activities rely to some extent on the expertise available in national universities. Again, many universities in developing countries have some capacity both specifically in nutrition and in other subjects of importance to surveillance. These are drawn upon to varying extents in most existing surveillance systems, mainly for design and for assistance in data analysis and interpretation. Here, too, opportunities can be sought to bring in the required expertise.

Resources and staffing needed

Since nutritional surveillance is always a part of other larger organizations, it is very difficult to assess the resources required. This depends very much on the extent to which existing facilities are used; where this is done extensively the additional resources required are not very great. However, a crucial question when considering nutritional surveillance is "how much is it going to cost?" – and some attempt should be made to give an approximate figure. The requirements should obviously be seen in the light of possible benefits. These in turn relate to the decisions that that will be taken in the light of the information provided by the surveillance system, and that should lead to more effective allocation of resources to improve nutrition. In the first instance, therefore, some approximate estimate may be needed; but before deciding on whether the cost is likely to be worth while, some rather careful calculations of the possible effects of an investment in information should be made.

The major additional requirement in terms of resources when establishing nutritional surveillance will usually be staff for the central unit. As a rough guide, a realistic minimum is perhaps about five professional staff assigned to the running of the programme and to analysis. As discussed earlier, the nutrition information system in Costa Rica has some twenty professionals engaged in the central unit; in Kenya two or three people are usually assigned at any one time to work specifically on nutrition but they are dependent on the much larger staff of the statistics bureau itself; the pilot project in Cali, Colombia, has about five professionals involved, and indeed this figure does seem to be near the minimum. No surveillance programme has any substantial number of field staff assigned *full-time* to nutritional surveillance. The practice is always to draw upon employees of other agencies. However, under some circumstances it may be worth considering employing some field staff, at least in a supervisory capacity. Alternatively, it may be possible to buy the time of people who are already assigned to the field.

Another major requirement is for training. This applies to training in data collection methods, as well as in managing the system in terms of data flow, and in data analysis and interpretation. Often, as discussed earlier, this will be part of the job of the staff of the central unit. The resources of affiliated institutions, including nutritional institutions, may be drawn upon for this.

The physical requirements for a surveillance system are: measuring equipment; forms and questionnaires; training materials; data-handling facilities, including computer time; and publications. The cost of equipment is small – cheap weighing scales are becoming widely available and are usually satisfactory; height boards for measuring children can be constructed relatively cheaply. These are the only additional pieces of equipment normally required. A device for measuring the heights of schoolchildren, consisting of a cardboard measuring strip and instructions, has been used in Costa Rica and can be transmitted through the mail. The cost of this is approximately US$ 1 per device.

Forms and questionnaires need to be developed, but the actual cost of their printing and distribution would not be great. Similarly, training materials will need to be developed, but the cost of distribution is again small. Computer time is likely to be a fairly major item. For operations within the government service, it may be possible to make use of spare capacity. None the less, it is extremely important to budget adequately for computer time and not to rely heavily on favours; it is much better to ensure that there is access to data processing as a business-like arrangement. Further, the need for computer time is generally underestimated, and sufficient allowance must be made.

Finally, the information needs to be disseminated in the form of reports, graphical presentations, maps, etc. The impact of information can be substantially enhanced by effective presentation. In particular, mapping is a useful device, and should be included when budgeting. Regular publications will cost a certain amount of money.

Transport has not been included in these estimates; this depends entirely on local availability. As with any other programme in developing countries, the ability to get about is an absolute necessity. This is particularly so in nutritional surveillance where field operations will need to be supported. Further, the surveillance unit itself must be able to investigate field problems, carry out periodic studies of its own, and so on. It may be that transport facilities should be budgeted for.

All in all, a nutritional surveillance programme when budgeted is similar to other programmes concerned with information and planning. Roughly 50-70% of the budget will probably be needed for staff. Experience shows that surveillance programmes do take some time to become fully operational, and a programme of at least 3–5 years' duration should be envisaged. As stressed earlier, the first phase should be an initial assessment, and during this the probable costs and outputs of the system should be assessed. What needs to be avoided, however, is expecting too much for too little. Probably it is only worth setting up a surveillance programme when sufficient resources can be made available to hire or assign the minimum number of five or so staff on a full-time basis.

REFERENCES

1. VALVERDE, V. ET AL. The organization of an information system for food and nutrition programmes in Costa Rica. *Food and nutrition*, **7**: 32-40 (1981).

2. *The Philippine Nutrition Program 1978-1982*. Manila, National Nutrition Council, 1977.

3. TRISTAN, M. Estudios antropológicos de clasificación funcional. *Boletín informativo del SIN*, No. 6, 24-32 (1980).

4. GUERRA, Q. A. Estudios antropológicos de clasificación funcional: análisis comparativo del poder adquistivo del salario del obrero bananero. *Boletín informativo del SIN*, **2** (10): 11-16 (1981).

5. National health information systems in South-East Asia. *WHO Chronicle*, **33**: 177-179 (1979).

6. Seminar on national health information systems. *WHO Chronicle,* **33**: 338-342 (1979).

7. WHO Technical Report Series, No. 472, 1971 *(Statistical indicators for the planning and evaluation of public health programmes. Fourteenth report of the WHO Expert Committee on Health Statistics).*

8. UNITED NATIONS. DEPARTMENT OF INTERNATIONAL ECONOMIC AND SOCIAL AFFAIRS. STATISTICAL OFFICE. *Studies in the integration of social statistics: technical report.* New York, United Nations, 1979 (Studies in Methods, Series F, No. 24; ST/ESA/STAT/SER. F/24).

CHAPTER 4

Nutritional surveillance for health and development planning: data characteristics, outputs, and sources

Summary

The characteristics of the data required for nutritional surveillance are determined by the causes of malnutrition, as expressed by the relationship between resources, their flow, and the nutritional and health outcome. Outcome indicators in common use are nutritional status (including low birth weight), infant and child mortality rates, morbidity, and measures of socioeconomic status and environmental health. Resource indicators are used to examine causes of malnutrition and to define population groups; they apply both at the village level (e.g., access to services, ecology, agricultural pattern) and at the level of the household (e.g., occupation, cropping pattern). Resource indicators offer many parallels with standard-of-living indicators and several of the latter (economic status, environmental sanitation, access to services) are identical with those used in nutritional surveillance. Flow indicators (production–income–expenditure–consumption) are more difficult to obtain and have a more limited role. The usual formats for data presentation involve the tabulation of indicators by population group. The use of a series of indicators is convenient for summarizing information. Some standardization of formats is proposed.

The general requirements for reliable indicators are that they should show relevance and disaggregation and should be susceptible to time-series analysis. There should also be reasonable certainty that they are representative and the selective testing of the significance of differences or association between indicators is desirable. Examples are given of data outputs and their interpretation in several countries.

The data are obtained either from administrative sources or from household surveys. They are usually available from government agencies and, in deciding which to use, trade-offs between availability, relevance, and cost become necessary. Most systems use health data from clinics. The education system is another potentially useful source of nutritional data. The usefulness of agricultural data for nutritional surveillance needs to be further explored. Local government administrations can provide data on vital statistics (births and deaths) and on village infrastructures and services. Censuses provide information on the sizes of population groups and on certain outcome variables. Community weighing programmes, in common with other sources of screening data, are also of potential value in nutritional surveillance. Data from household budget surveys can sometimes be interpreted to derive indicators of food consumption. Moreover, the collection of anthropometric data can be added (as a "nutrition module") to household surveys, thus providing a useful source of nutritional data linked with socioeconomic and agricultural variables.

Data Characteristics and Outputs

In Chapter 1, we introduced the concept of resources and outcome, the two being linked by a flow of events (see Fig. 1.1), and noted that this concept helps to define the variables needed for nutritional surveillance. Resource and outcome variables are relatively stable, and their values can often be measured objectively – they tend to be referred to in terms of "status" (economic, health, nutritional, etc.). The flow of events varies more rapidly, and its measurement at one point in time is less easy to make and interpret. The measurement of resources and outcome is, in practice, treated differently from that of flow.

Variables that measure resources and outcome are of particular interest in nutritional surveillance. **Resource** variables describe different population groups by, for example, agro-ecological zone, type of farming system, cropping pattern, access to services, etc. They are mainly used as descriptive factors for classifying groups, and hence also for explaining differences in outcome variables between groups. **Outcome** variables include nutritional status, morbidity and mortality; factors associated with these biological variables, for example, sanitation and housing, are also included, essentially as "proxies" for exposure to infectious diseases and income. Such variables tend to change relatively slowly, which has the advantage that a single measurement can reflect conditions over a substantial preceding period. Certain measurements (e.g., nutritional status, housing) also have the advantage of being obtainable by direct observation or measurement.

Flow variables – production, distribution, income, expenditure, consumption – account for the links between resources and outcome, as represented in Fig. 1.1. Information on them is needed for projections of future changes in food consumption; it is not essential for describing nutritional conditions at one point in time or for monitoring changes in outcome. Flow variables are not often included in nutritional surveillance systems, since they are more difficult to collect accurately than resource or outcome data, and the values change more rapidly (week-to-week, seasonally). Where recall methods based on question-naires are used, repeated visits are desirable, and it is difficult to check responses objectively. Those variables that can be physically measured present substantial difficulties in the field: in many cases, crop-cutting and area measurements for production estimates are rendered problematic by traditional agricultural practices; similarly, estimates of food consumption by weighing demand a lot of time from well-trained enumerators.

To recapitulate, the information produced from nutritional surveillance systems for health and development planning aims at answering the questions in Table 3.1: Which groups are most affected by malnutrition and what are their characteristics? How is this situation changing for specific groups, and why? Are specific problems indicated? And, in the light of the answers to all these, what should be done? The basic outputs are tabulations of outcome indicators by relevant socioeconomic or geographical group. The indicators most widely used are: anthropometric measurements of nutritional status, health data, socioeconomic data, and environmental data. Biological indicators of wide application can be identified from experience; these are not very culture-specific since the basic biology is the same for all populations. The choice of socioeconomic and environmental indicators depends much more on individual circumstances and on opportunities for using available data.

For many uses, the precise choice of outcome indicator is not the most pressing problem, at least to begin with. It seems to be better, within limits, to

Table 4.1. Summary of outputs of selected surveillance systems

System	Data collected	Periodicity	Level of aggregation	Output available	Circulated to
CHILE					
Conpan (1)	Weight, age	(1) Monthly	(1) By clinic	(1) Graphs of monthly prevalences by clinic	Health and other ministries
Sivide (2)	Vital statistics, including birth weight; Presenting illnesses; Coverage and delivery of services	(2) Yearly	(2) Regional and national	(2) Cross-tabulations of single indicators; cross-sectional by region, time series on national basis	
COLOMBIA					
Pilot system at state level	Incidence of infectious disease	Monthly	Health centre/county	Maps, descending ranking in sextiles	Monthly reports to health centres, hospitals, national and regional planning offices. Colombian Institute of Family Welfare, universities, etc. Time-series data on morbidity circulated to central health offices.
	Mortality	4-monthly	County	Some time-series graphs	
	Coverage of immunization	Monthly	Health centre/county	As above + histograms	
	Birth weight	Monthly			
	Ht/Age, Wt/Age, Wt/Ht	4-monthly			
	Crops, hectares planted, harvested, yield, price, farm wages, available protein, calories	6-monthly	County	Ranking in sextiles, maps, % change over previous semester	

	Data characteristics	Frequency	Disaggregation	Outputs	Sources
COSTA RICA National (SIN)	School heights	2-yearly	District-canton-province region-subregion	Height retardation, infant mortality, birth-weights by district, canton, province region and subregion	Min. of Labour, Min. of Development, Family Allowances Programme, Min. of Health, Min. of Agriculture, Min. of Planning
	Wt, age all children < 6 yrs	Yearly			
	Vaccinations				
	Family planning reports				
	Sanitation reports				
	Occupation/landholding	2-yearly	Family/rural health community	Distribution of functional groups in ten counties, social and economic characteristics	
	Migration				
	Housing	Yearly			
EL SALVADOR	Wt, age	6-monthly	Urban/rural	Prevalences IInd, IIIrd degree (Gomez)	Ministries
KENYA Integrated rural surveys plus nutrition module	Wt/Ht, Ht/Age, Wt/Age ages 1 through 5	3-monthly to yearly, 2-yearly for nutritional status	Province Agro-zone Income group Land holding	Cross tabulations of indicators	Sectors, Ministry of Planning
	Descriptive variables				
	Farm production				
	Income				
	Access to services				
	Occupation, etc.				
PHILIPPINES National weighing programme	0-6 yrs Wt, age	6-monthly	Village Municipality Province Region	Prevalences Ist, IInd, IIIrd (Gomez) (local standards)	Municipal, regional, provincial planners Municipal health clinics
SRI LANKA	Height, age All children entering primary school	Yearly	School, village, estate	Table showing % below 80% Wt/Age by province, under 5 pop., clinic enrolment, % pop. seen	Food & Nutrition, Policy Planning Division of the Ministry of Plan Implementation
	Birth weights	Monthly	Hospital, clinic, MOH division		

concentrate at first on using data that are available or can be readily obtained rather than put further resources into collecting additional data. Often it has been possible to reach similar conclusions, using, say, weight-for-age (Wt/Age) of preschool children, or height-for-age (Ht/Age) of schoolchildren, or child mortality rates, because in practice these indicators are often fairly closely associated with each other within population groups. Nutritional surveillance has begun by making use of the data at hand and then moving on to more deliberately selected indicators. For example, the surveillance programme in Costa Rica and the Philippines started with patchy anthropometric data on preschool children – because these were available from the health system – and subsequently obtained more precise information with greater coverage through a survey of schoolchildren's heights.

A summary of outputs from selected surveillance systems is given in Table 4.1. Indicators derived from anthropometric measurements are common to all the examples. In certain cases, these are the only indicators analysed at present. In others, health data and, infrequently, food availability and socioeconomic data are available. These are usually presented as cross-tabulations of single indicators. The following sections give some details on outputs from surveillance systems based on different types of indicator.

Outcome variables

The usual measurements of nutritional outcome are nutritional status of children (including prevalence of low birth weight), infant and child mortality rates, and prevalences of infectious diseases. Certain environmental and socioeconomic data are also sometimes treated as outcome indicators.

Nutritional status

~ Three important indicators of nutritional status are used in surveillance, and all are also considered to be indicators of health status (*1*, p. 18):

— anthropometric measurements of preschool children
— heights (and sometimes weights) of children at school entry
— prevalence of low birth weight (less than 2.5 kg).

The commonest anthropometric measurements of preschool children are of weight and height, combined with age. The age range is often from 6 months to 5 years in sample surveys; frequently, however, younger infants are also included, as are children up to 7 years. The selection, collection, and analysis of these measurements are extensively covered in the literature (see, for example, ref. *2* and *3*). Since a great deal of emphasis is placed on anthropometric measurements of children in nutritional surveillance, some further explanation is given below. Where a high proportion of births take place in clinics or health centres, birth weights are frequently recorded and may be used to give indicators of the prevalence of low birth weight. Where they represent a high proportion of the population, schoolchildren are a potentially important source of anthropometric data; while such data do not reflect immediate problems of malnutrition, they are important as long-term indicators of nutritional conditions.

Infants and preschool children

Birth weights of babies delivered in health centres or at attended deliveries are recorded and used in several surveillance systems. The indicator normally used is the percentage of babies with a birth weight below 2.5 kg. This indicator is obviously most useful when a substantial proportion of births are attended, and the problem is that it is often not well known how far this is so. Differences between birth weights in different occupational groups have been observed in Costa Rica.[1] In Colombia, increases in food prices have been linked with an increased proportion of low birth weight babies three months later (L. Fajardo, personal communication, 1981).

Anthropometric data on preschool children are the main outcome indicator in most surveillance programmes. It may be useful to explain some of their advantages at this point. They are readily analysed by geographical area and socioeconomic group (see below), and can be shown to be related to determining factors such as income, environmental sanitation, and wealth. They are therefore a convenient means of defining relative nutritional conditions in different groups. Moreover, they permit changes over time to be assessed. Many other methods have been used at various times to describe the nutritional condition of individuals and populations: for example, food balance sheets, food consumption surveys, clinical examinations, and biochemical tests. Anthropometric measurements indicate the combined impact of factors affecting food availability at the household level (e.g., income, prices, national or local production, and marketing), the level of food consumption by particular individuals within a family (as determined by food habits, time at mother's disposal, mother's level of education and knowledge of the nutritional value of foods), and the child's health record, itself a resultant of environmental influences. Anthropometric measurements thus provide a logical endpoint (with mortality rates) to the sequence of events shown in Fig. 1.1.

Biochemical and clinical indicators may provide the same kind of information to some extent. Clinical observations of protein-energy malnutrition are significant for serious cases, where there is severe wasting and/or oedema. For more moderate cases, anthropometry (especially over time, e.g., using growth, or "road-to-health" charts) is in any case the best means of clinical assessment, and it is also necessary for quantifying wasting, even when this is severe. Biochemical data are mainly useful in connection with micronutrient deficiencies; serum protein or albumin levels are useful for research into protein-energy

---

[1] BERMÚDEZ, M. A. Factores relacionados con el peso al nacer, Costa Rica, 1976-1977. Informe del Sistema de Información en Nutrición, noviembre. San José, Oficina de Información, Casa Presidencial, 1980, p. 44.

malnutrition, but are hardly essential for surveillance. Surveys involving the collection of clinical and biochemical measurements are expensive, since they require medical personnel, whereas anthropometric measurements can be taken by nonmedical enumerators. Well-tested procedures for standardizing anthropometric measurements are available (4).

Anthropometric measurements have been shown to predict mortality risk. For example, the Pan American study of mortality in childhood revealed the relative importance of growth retardation as a cause of mortality in children (5). Other studies in Bangladesh (6, 7) and India (8) have confirmed this.

Controversy has arisen in the past about the use of growth patterns of children from developed countries to measure growth retardation in children from developing countries. As Habicht et al. (9) have shown, food intakes and health status are likely to be more important in explaining differences in attained anthropometric measurements than are possible genetic differences in growth potential. Children in elite groups in developing countries show growth patterns that are almost identical with international standards, at least up to the age of 5.

The anthropometric indicator most commonly used is weight-for-age (Wt/Age), the age range usually being 0–7 years, though 1–5 years is also frequent. Data are obtained both from surveys and from the health system. When data are derived from clinics or weighing programmes, only weight and age are usually available. Cut-off points are most often either based on the Gomez classification or taken as 60% and 80% Wt/Age. For the Gomez classification, widely used in Latin America, the cut-off points are 60%, 75%, and 90% (10). One reason for selecting the 75% or 80% value as the usual cut-off point is that, in a normally growing population of children, the value of the third percentile from 12 to 60 months of age ranges from 80% to 82.4% Wt/Age. Thus, only a small proportion of children are expected to show values below 75% or 80%.

The Wellcome classification (11) defines malnutrition using similar cut-off points: below 60% Wt/Age (without oedema) for marasmus, and between 60% and 80% Wt/Age for underweight. Survey measurements often include height, so that indicators based on weight-for-height (Wt/Ht) and height-for-age (Ht/Age) are also computed. For these, the cut-off points are usually 80% Wt/Ht and 90% Ht/Age. Results for Wt/Ht and Ht/Age are generally presented separately, although a division into four categories (normal, stunted not wasted, wasted not stunted, wasted and stunted), i.e., the Waterlow classification (12), has also been used (e.g., Sri Lanka, 13). This has the advantage of distinguishing between chronic and acute malnutrition. In planning for development, Ht/Age has probably proved the most useful means of measuring nutritional status (e.g., Kenya, 14, 15).

The reference growth data most widely used in determining Wt/Age, Ht/Age, and Wt/Ht values are those put forward by WHO (2), which are based on figures for reference populations studied by the US National Center for Health Statistics (NCHS) (16). National standards are used in certain surveillance programmes (e.g., Colombia (17); Philippines (18, pp. 31-32)).

School-age children

Indicators based on heights of schoolchildren have been derived in Costa Rica from a school census. Data were presented in terms of percentages of children with heights less than 90% of the median heights of children of the same age and sex in the Iowa reference population – defined as height retardation – by districts, cantons, and provinces (administrative divisions) and/or by regional and subregional divisions used by government agencies (*19, 20*).

In countries where school enrolment is high, height retardation (e.g., among first-graders) is a promising indicator. This is particularly so when the heights of schoolchildren are routinely measured at school, in which case tabulations of schoolchildren's heights are often to be found in local education offices. Probably on a sample basis, these need to be analysed to give relative levels of height retardation in different groups and to follow long-term changes.

Examples of outputs of anthropometric data

In Costa Rica, data from available anthropometric and socioeconomic surveys have been analysed by income group and occupational group, as shown in Table 4.2. Routinely collected birth-weight data have also been analysed for several years[1] by province and, as shown in Table 4.3, by father's occupational group. Data from the first survey of heights of children entering the first grade of school have been presented, by region and subregion, and also linked to socioeconomic conditions as ascertained from housing and population censuses at the cantonal level, which will be discussed later (see Table 4.16). The results shown in these three tables illustrate several important points. They indicate, by administrative area and by occupation, which groups are most affected by malnutrition and show that there is a good case for focusing on these groups, both for economy of effort and because of their special importance.

Baseline data (or data interpreted at one point in time) such as these have policy implications that may be important and usable before time-series data become available (see question 1 in Table 3.1). The regular collection of such data would provide certain of the outputs needed from a surveillance system – the intervals could be of the order of two years or possibly more (see question 2 in Table 3.1). However, the replication of these data alone might not fully meet surveillance needs, in at least two related respects: (1), the use of additional outcome variables aids interpretation since the movement of a few related indicators together (or not) makes for greater insight and a broader application; (2) additional data e.g., data on programme delivery could make it possible to use the results for evaluation (see also Chapter 6).

---

[1] BERMÚDEZ, M. A. *Factores relacionados con el peso al nacer, Costa Rica, 1976-1977. Informe del Sistema de Información en Nutrición, noviembre*. San José, Oficina de Información, Casa Presidencial, 1980.

Table 4.2. Percentage of children in Costa Rica
in different weight-for-age categories according to father's occupation [a]

Occupation of father	No. of cases	Percentage of children in weight-for-age (Gomez) category					
		Normal	First degree	Second degree	Third degree	Second and third degree	Total
Labourers in sugar-cane plantations	30	33.3	46.6	20.0	0.1	20.1	100.0
Labourers in banana plantations	86	44.2	38.4	16.3	1.1	17.4	100.0
Farmers in staple grain farms	107	43.9	43.0	12.2	0.9	13.1	100.0
Labourers in cattle ranches	96	40.6	46.9	12.5	0.0	12.5	100.0
Farmers in coffee farms	81	53.1	34.6	11.1	1.2	12.3	100.0
Unemployed	164	50.6	39.0	10.4	0.0	10.4	100.0
Labourers in farms dedicated to other agricultural products	79	53.2	36.7	6.3	3.8	10.1	100.0
Labourers in staple grain farms	42	47.6	42.9	9.5	0.0	9.5	100.0
Labourers in coffee farms	44	45.4	45.4	9.2	0.0	9.2	100.0
Labourers in African palm plantations	23	43.5	47.8	8.7	0.0	8.7	100.0
Non-agricultural workers	889	56.5	35.2	7.9	0.4	8.3	100.0
Labourers in dairy products	40	67.5	25.0	7.5	0.0	7.5	100.0
Farmers in farms dedicated to other agricultural products	66	65.1	28.8	6.1	0.0	6.1	100.0
Farmers in cattle ranches	38	50.0	50.0	0.0	0.0	0.0	100.0
Other occupations	26	61.5	38.5	0.0	0.0	0.0	100.0

[a] Adapted from ref. 47.

Table 4.3. Distribution of birth weights in Costa Rica according to father's occupation [a]

Occupation of father	Weight at birth		
	Low	Normal	Overweight
Professionals	5.1	90.2	4.7
Managers and administrators	5.7	88.9	5.4
Salesmen	6.0	88.9	5.1
Other craftsmen	6.1	89.0	4.9
Office workers	6.7	89.0	4.3
Agricultural workers	6.8	88.8	4.4
Bus drivers, taxi drivers, etc.	6.8	87.9	5.2
Craftsmen	6.9	88.8	4.3
Students	7.2	89.4	3.5
Privately employed labourers	7.5	88.6	4.0
Domestic workers	7.7	82.1	10.3
Unskilled labourers	8.5	87.8	3.7
Poorly specified [b]	7.4	88.3	4.3

[a] Source: Bermúdez, M. *Factores relacionados con el peso al nacer, Costa Rica, 1976-1977. Informe del Sistema de Información en Nutrición, noviembre.* San José, Oficina de Información, Casa Presidencial, 1980, p. 44.
[b] Includes the crippled (55).

The use of results from clinics depends to a great extent on their timing. Monthly changes in three of the eight clinics covered by the Consultorios Sensores system in Chile are shown in Fig. 4.1. These data are more finely focused than national and regional data, both in time and geographically. The following points can be made about such information. It leads to more rapid conclusions on overall trends than annually aggregated data, though these conclusions are tentative. Here, a trend towards improvement is apparent after the analysis of only 18 months' data for all three clinics, despite monthly variations, while in the case of clinic B, where data for three years were analysed, the improvement is particularly marked. Such information also shows whether changes are likely to be local or general and what seasonal changes there are. Thus the detection of a seasonal peak for all eight clinics demonstrates that some additional or modified effort may be needed in the latter part of each year.

Other uses of such data depend on timing. If they become available within a month or so of their collection, they could be used to initiate action in response to a deterioration in the situation. This would require (*a*) a mechanism for initiating action, and (*b*) prior decisions on the indicator levels at which such action should be taken (see also Chapter 6 on timely warning and intervention programmes). On the other hand, data presented with several months' delay still have their uses, though these are different. They would still show that seasonal changes occur and give an earlier indication of trends than, say, annual figures;

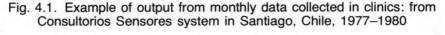

Fig. 4.1. Example of output from monthly data collected in clinics: from Consultorios Sensores system in Santiago, Chile, 1977–1980

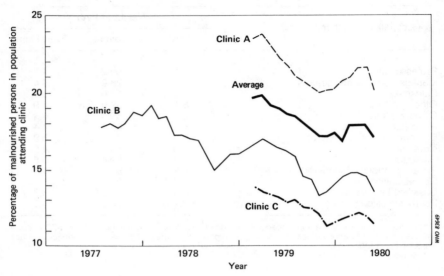

however, decisions on interventions and resource allocations would tend to be relatively long-term and essentially concerned with setting targets in both geographical and temporal terms.

Anthropometric data in Kenya were obtained through the inclusion of a nutrition module in the continuing Integrated Rural Surveys. Data collection was carried out in two rounds, one completed in November 1977, and the other from October 1978 to February 1979. The results are shown by province and by agro-ecological zone in Table 4.4. This is one of the few available examples of national time-series data. The results by province provide a good example of the conventional output to be expected from a surveillance system based on the collection of sample data.

The groupings show that differences in nutritional status at any one moment may also provide evidence of nutritional changes over time; this would be so when the definition of groups is related to those factors that cause changes in nutritional conditions. In the data here, this seems to have been the case. This type of breakdown was originally found useful in the case of the 1977 data, as a means of highlighting differences in child nutrition by area. In two agrozones (numbers 7 and 8) important changes in nutritional status were detected between 1977 and 1979. There was drought in these areas for two or more years prior to 1977, after which conditions became more favourable. The results may there-fore reflect the effects of past droughts, suggesting that the malnutrition in this area was due to the frequent droughts as much as to other predisposing factors

Table 4.4. Changes in nutritional status in Kenya, 1977–1979 [a]

A. Agro-ecological zones

	1	2	3	4	5	6	7	8	10/11	Mean, population weighted
% Population	13	15	19	7	15	5	11	9	6	
%<90% Ht/Age										
1977	21	21	30	25	35	28	44	40	20	29.6
1979	25	27	27	21	26	31	20	19	40	25.7
%<80% Wt/Ht										
1977	4	6	3	3	3	8	6	3	9	4.5
1979	2	2	4	4	2	0	3	3	6	2.9
Changes Ht/Age %<90%	+4	+6	-3	-4	-9	+3	-24	-21	+20	-2.5
Changes Wt/Ht %<80%	-2	-4	+1	+1	-1	-8	-3	0	-3	-1.7

B. Provinces

	Central	Coast	Eastern	Nyanza	Rift Valley	Western	Mean
%<80% Wt/Age 1977	39	24	41	24	34	27	33
%<80% Wt/Age 1979	23	29	29	27	27	21	26
Changes Wt/Age %<80%	-16	+5	-12	+3	-7	-6	-7

[a] Abbreviations: Ht/Age = Height-for-age, Wt/Ht = Weight-for-height, Wt/Age = Weight-for-age; %<90% etc. refer to less than 90% of Harvard Standard. Calculations based on the figures given in ref. 14 and 15.

(e.g., land pressure or soil fertility); in this case, the vulnerability of the area to drought would require attention, the existing measures being apparently ineffective.

The anthropometric changes observed in agrozone 7 also suggest that it might be advantageous to use multiple indicators. If a series of indicators was available, these would serve to check the consistency of the results. For example, a housing indicator (or some other long-term measure of socioeconomic status) would change relatively slowly and provide a check on the comparability of samples; rainfall, production figures, and prices might show movements credibly related to observed nutritional changes; and morbidity and mortality figures could confirm conclusions on outcome.

Infant and child mortality rates

Registers of births and deaths may be used to obtain data on general mortality, infant mortality, and mortality rates for children aged 1–4 years. Problems of coverage and underreporting of deaths in certain areas may impose serious limitations on comparisons between regions or on analyses of mortality changes over time. None the less, where available, mortality rates offer perhaps the most fundamental indicators of all. These rates are also difficult to assess accurately in sample surveys. For precise information (e.g., in the World Fertility Survey (21)), detailed fertility histories and records of living children have been considered necessary, and even then accurate information cannot be obtained in certain cultures. Indicators relating to child mortality rates have been obtained more simply by questionnaires concerning the numbers of live births mothers have had and the numbers of surviving children (57).

Infant and child mortality rates are used in most of the surveillance systems reviewed in Latin America, though nowhere else at present. The usual indicators are annual mortality rates for infants and young children expressed as deaths per 1000 live births and per 1000 population aged 1–4 years, respectively, and are analysed by administrative area or nationally. Data from Colombia are analysed on a monthly basis, by cause of death, at municipal level. Similar data are available at national and regional levels from the other Latin American countries, on an annual or biannual basis; this frequency is suitable as regards the use of the data.

Morbidity rates

The health system often provides information on the prevalence of infectious diseases which is derived from data collected at clinics. Prevalences of infectious diseases in children can also be assessed in household surveys by means of questionnaires asking mothers whether a child has had fever or diarrhoea in the previous 1–7 days (e.g., Egypt (22)). This approach is still somewhat experimental in cross-sectional surveys, although it is accepted practice in longitudinal studies.

Information on prevalences of common infectious diseases, generally with reference to children, is included in the surveillance systems in Chile, Colombia, Costa Rica, and certain Central American countries. The diseases covered are much the same as in the case of health information systems. In many other countries, data of this kind derived from routine ministry of health operations could be included in surveillance systems. The basic data on morbidity are generally in the form of weekly, monthly, or quarterly summaries, by administrative area.

Immunization rates are reported, monthly and by municipality, in Colombia; in Costa Rica, reports by community are provided every six months, then aggregated.

Examples of health and mortality data

Data are available from Chile showing infant mortality rates at the national level over a number of years, (see Table 4.5). These can be broken down, for example, by occupational group and education (see Table 4.6). Similar data have been produced by administrative areas in Costa Rica; these are also available on a time basis (see Fig. 3.6). Figures showing a trend such as that in Table 4.5 should be of special interest both to ministries of health and to those in government who are more generally concerned with living standards and social welfare. The data presented show a steady improvement, which must level out some time in the future. Failure to improve or deterioration would also be picked up by such data.

Mortality rates used at one point in time permit useful comparisons between areas or socioeconomic groups (see Table 4.6). Regional data allow regions with priority needs to be identified. Analysis of the results by region over time extends the picture. Apart from regularly confirming or modifying priorities through cross-sectional analyses, such time-series data would indicate whether a general improvement observed nationally was occurring in all regions (i.e., would answer questions 2 (*b*) and 2 (*c*) in Table 3.1). If certain regions were lagging behind, the causes might be assessed and the necessary measures identified.

Comparisons between different occupational groups, as in Table 4.6, give information on priorities but with different implications regarding targets and policy. While regional targeting may be desirable in the case of nutritional or public health programmes, reaching distinct socioeconomic groups is an important consideration when development policies and programmes are being designed.

One example of the reporting of infectious disease within a nutritional surveillance programme comes from the pilot project in Valle del Cauca, Colombia. The use of such data is crucially dependent on the timing of the reporting. In this instance, results are reported within a month of collection and early assessments are made available informally when there are indications of an outbreak of the disease. Action is then taken to control the outbreak.

Table 4.5. Infant mortality rates (per 1000 live births) in Chile, 1930–1978 [a]

	1930	1940	1950	1960	1965	1968	1969	1970
Rate	234	192	136	126	100	83.5	78.7	79.3

	1971	1972	1973	1974	1975	1976	1977	1978
Rate	70.5	71.1	65.2	63.3	55.4	54.0	47.5	38.7

[a] Based on ref. 48, p. 18 and 49, p. 11.

Table 4.6. Infant mortality rates in Chile according to father's occupation, educational level of mother, and birth order: birth cohorts from 1972 (rates per 1000 live births) [a]

Occupation of father and education of mother	Total	Birth order					
		1	2	3	4	5	≥6
Employed	29.8	23.4	27.1	32.4	41.1	48.0	52.5
None	84.3	68.7	54.2	85.5	111.1	133.3	118.4
Primary	38.1	29.5	38.1	41.6	40.1	52.2	49.2
Secondary and higher	23.8	20.2	21.3	25.7	40.2	37.8	51.4
Workers	66.9	59.1	66.0	65.6	67.9	71.9	77.8
None	108.6	126.2	131.5	107.2	114.7	101.5	97.1
Primary	62.7	57.2	62.0	61.8	63.2	65.4	71.6
Secondary and higher	59.9	48.6	62.8	65.3	53.9	101.2	105.9

[a] Source: ref. 50, p. 53.

Sanitary and socioeconomic environment

These variables are hybrid. They are determinants rather than measures of nutritional outcome. However, they change slowly, and are in a sense outcomes of the sequence of events, starting with resources and continuing through the production–income–expenditure–consumption flow, as shown in Fig. 1.1. They also serve as "proxies" for infection and income, respectively. Pragmatically, they have the important virtue of being rather simple to measure objectively. Their inclusion as outcome indicators is accordingly advocated, even if they do not fit as neatly into the concept as one might wish. Depending on the analytical requirements, they are also treated as descriptive variables for defining groups. The use of variables such as these as outcome indicators or for descriptive purposes depends on the planning needs, just as in statistical analyses variables are treated as dependent or independent according to the questions to be answered.

Sanitary environment can be assessed by such data as: type of water supply, distance to water (taking seasonal factors into account, if necessary), toilet facilities, and garbage disposal facilities. Such information is quite readily obtained by interview or direct observation. The socioeconomic environment or degree of wealth can be assessed by data such as: housing, ownership of consumer durables (and cattle, in some situations), and facilities for child education. These data are discussed further in the next section.

Resource variables

Indicators measuring resources are useful both for setting targets and, because by association they suggest what action may be needed, for formulating policies and programmes. In the cross-tabulations that form the main outputs for surveillance, outcome variables are presented by socioeconomic group defined by resource variables. This presentation is chosen because:

– certain groups may be of particular concern;
– differences in nutritional conditions are highlighted by this disaggregation;
– changes over time may be more apparent when related to specific groups, and also have more important policy implications;
– the targeting of measures both specific to nutrition (e.g., health and nutrition intervention programme) and non-specific (e.g., development programmes) and the monitoring of their impact represent an important set of decisions that have to be supported by surveillance.

These variables fall into two groups: those applying to villages or communities, and those applying to households. Most of them, particularly at the village or community level, are rather easy to determine from existing data or through interviews. Examples are:

Village or community variables: ecological zone; altitude and/or topography; accessibility (e.g., distance from road, nearest town, markets, etc. or time to reach these); climate; access to services (health, education, agricultural extension, cooperatives); cropping pattern, endemic diseases; water supply (if communal).

Household variables: occupation of household head and other income-earners; land-holding area; land-tenure status; access to credit; production inputs; farming system and cropping pattern; use of technology, fertilizer, other inputs; water supply; educational levels; etc.

Many of these variables are recorded in normal household surveys. They can quite readily be added to collections of nutritional data, particularly in the case of village/community variables, whether the data are obtained from administrative sources or from sample surveys. Often it is only possible to link data from different sources by area; this means that, for example, the prevalence of malnutrition may be available for one province from one source, and the percentage of unemployment for the same province from another source. Although linkages of such data are useful, they have much greater validity at lower levels of aggregation. Efforts to include resource variables for linkage, e.g., occupation, cropping pattern, etc., should have priority. These variables should be collected with respect to the items for which other data are available, i.e., children's parents, households, farms, etc.

Further details on resource variables are given later in Table 4.10, but first their clear relationship to level-of-living indicators, social statistics, "health for all" indicators, etc. needs to be brought out.

Nutritional surveillance and other indicator series

Other indicators in addition to nutritional status are of importance in nutritional surveillance because they may be associated with or causally related to nutritional outcome. Conversely, nutritional data are among the outputs used for assessing and monitoring "level of living", which may be variously expressed as basic needs, social indicators, welfare measurements, etc. It has also been noted that nutritional indicators are important health status indicators (1, p. 19). This means both that nutritional surveillance has a place in the context of social monitoring, and that concepts and experience in the field of social monitoring can be drawn on for nutritional surveillance purposes.

In the last decade, attention has largely shifted from reliance on national accounts of economic performance, notably in terms of GNP or GDP, towards other ways of measuring a society's performance (see, for example, ref. 23). Here are some examples:

– Social indicators as defined by the United Nations Statistical Office (UNSO) have been divided into 12 categories: population; family formation, families and households; learning and educational services; earning activities and the inactive; distribution of income, consumption, and accumulation; social security and welfare services; health services and nutrition; housing and its environment; public order and safety; time use; leisure and culture; social stratification and mobility (24). A typical example of a series of indicators for intercountry comparisons is given in Table 4.7.

– Welfare-oriented measurements have been proposed to supplement national accounts; for our purposes, the most relevant here are the measurement of assets, categorized as: tangible reproducible assets (e.g., buildings, equipment, consumer durables); tangible non-reproducible assets (e.g., natural resources, land); intangible non-financial assets (human capital and knowledge, possibly including health); financial assets (23).

– Basic needs indicators are used by ILO. Those mentioned in *Basic needs performance* (25), include: calorie consumption; access to water; life expectancy; deaths due to disease; literacy; doctors and nurses per population; rooms per person; GNP per capita.

– Certain indicators have been proposed for evaluating progress towards "health for all" (1): these are shown in Table 4.8. Again, the relationship with nutritional surveillance is clear: a nutritional surveillance system can provide information for health monitoring; on the other hand, a health information system provides information for nutritional surveillance.

Certain of these indicators can be selected for attention in surveillance programmes. This will create an overlap between nutritional surveillance and social and health monitoring – or an integration, depending on the approach taken. Nutritional surveillance outputs, disaggregated to refer to population groups within countries, should look something like Table 4.7. Certain additional indicators, particularly anthropometric and health indicators, can be added. Further outcome indicators that are widely used include: socioeconomic status (i.e., wealth, assets); environment, notably health environment; access to services; education. Nutritional surveillance and social indicator systems are compared in Table 4.9. They differ mainly in emphasis and should eventually become integrated.

Table 4.9 shows that most of the indicators that have so far been considered are already of concern outside the immediate perspective of nutrition. The absence of nutritional status (anthropometric) data from certain series may be due more to lack of data than to lack of relevance. The use of food consumption data must also be mentioned: the figures used (e.g., in Table 4.7) are derived from food balance-sheet calculations (for the United Nations table, a calculation based on distributions was evidently used) and may not be of much use in more disaggregated form. There is obviously no need for a country to adopt a whole series of different indicator (or "surveillance") systems. Within reason, they could all be part of one national system. In considering the possible contribution of nutritional surveillance, two particular points may be borne in mind. First, nutrition is a meeting-point of many of the different areas involved, so it can form an integrating focus. Secondly, the surveillance concept goes beyond the mere collection of data and emphasizes that only information needed for action should be obtained.

Procedures for establishing nutritional surveillance and the development of social and health statistics will in practice be interdependent. Where such statistics are routinely collected, the development of nutritional surveillance may start by introducing nutritional measurements into the existing system and strengthening it. In other circumstances nutrition itself may be the starting-point, and the utility of the nutritional surveillance system may be enhanced by

Table 4.7. Indicators of living conditions in groups of countries at di

Country group [c]	Health and nutrition						
	Percentage of population with calorie intake below critical limit, 1974	Life expectancy at birth, 1970-1975	Infant mortality, 1970-1975	Population per physician, 1975	Population per hospital bed, 1975	Access to community water supply [d]	F
						Percentage of urban population, 1975	Percentage of rural population, 1975
	1	2	3	4	5	6	7
I. Countries with per capita GDP in 1970 of less than $200	35	44	119	19 000	690	69	15
II. Countries with per capita GDP in 1970 of $200 or more but less than $400	20	52	76	3 700	480	88	18
III. Countries with per capita GDP in 1970 of $400 or more but less than $1000	15	61	51	2 000	260	91	55
IV. Countries with per capita GDP in 1970 of $1000 and more	—	71	19	670	105	—	—
V. Centrally planned economies of Eastern Europe and USSR	—	70	33	520	120	—	—

[a] Source: Centre for Development Planning, Projections and Policies, Department of International Economic a Affairs of the United Nations Secretariat, based on various international sources (52, p. 36).
[b] The figures presented here are medians.
[c] Centrally planned economies, for which gross domestic product data are not available, are shown as a separa Because of lack of information, the number of countries covered in the present table varies from indicator to indicator. indicator the number of countries is as follows: column 1: 55; columns 2 and 3: 101; column 4: 115; column 5: 125; 64; column 7: 50; column 8: 51; columns 9, 10 and 11: 119; column 12: 83.

providing social information to persons in government with data needs broader than nutrition alone. This is precisely what happened in Costa Rica with the *Sistema de Información en Nutrición (SIN)*, which was created as the starting-point for a more comprehensive national information system.

Common status indicators.

Many indicators useful for nutritional surveillance may already be available. A list of indicators commonly used to measure level of living will be found in Table 4.10; some details on them are given below.

of development, latest available year [a,b]

	Education					
	Enrolment ratio, 1974 [e]				Adult literacy ratio, c.1970 [f]	Country group [c]
level	Second level		Third level			
Female	Total	Female	Total	Female		
9	10		11		12	
43	11	6	0.6	0.2	19	I. Countries with per capita GDP in 1970 of less than $200
80	26	20	4.0	2.3	50	II. Countries with per capita GDP in 1970 of $200 or more but less than $400
106	51	51	7.7	5.0	84	III. Countries with per capita GDP in 1970 of $400 or more but less than $1000
103	75	73	20	16	99	IV. Countries with per capita GDP in 1970 of $1000 and more
100	56	56	16	13	—	V. Centrally planned economies of Eastern Europe and USSR

entage of urban population served by house connexion or public standposts, and percentage of rural population with
e access to water.
ber of students enrolled as a percentage of the total population in the age group corresponding to the three levels of
.
er of persons knowing how to read and write as a percentage of the total population in the age group 15 years and

Economic status indicators summarize long-term economic activity retroactively over a substantial period. In effect, therefore, they measure the stock of assets, or wealth. A list of indicators of economic status, which were taken from the social indicators proposed by the United Nations and which should be considered for inclusion in nutritional surveillance systems, is given in Table 4.10, section 1. Exact definitions (e.g., percentage of persons occupying living quarters with 3 or more persons per room) are given in the relevant document of the United Nations Statistical Office (24). Many of the indicators are more or less widely used for their own specific purposes (e.g., housing to

Table 4.8. Indicators proposed
for monitoring progress towards health for all [a]

---

(1) Health policy indicators:
— political commitment to health for all
— resource allocation
— the degree of equity of distribution of health resources
— community involvement in attaining health for all
— organizational framework and managerial process

(2) Social and economic indicators related to health:
— rate of population increase
— gross national product or gross domestic product
— income distribution
— work conditions
— adult literacy rate
— housing
— food availability

(3) Indicators of the provision of health care:
— coverage by primary health care
— coverage by the referral system

(4) Health status indicators:
— nutritional status and psychosocial development of children
— infant mortality rate
— child mortality rate (ages 1–4 years inclusive)
— life expectancy at birth or at other specific ages
— maternal mortality rate

---

[a] Source: WHO (*1*, p. 18).

measure housing itself, rather than economic status). The existence of major surveys in these areas (see, for example, ref. *26* and *27*) testifies to the availability of such data.

Environmental variables of interest in nutritional surveillance are given in Table 4.10, section 2. These are all familiar and quite commonly reported, and their likely association with nutrition and health is obvious. One example of a data output is furnished by columns 6, 7 and 8 of Table 4.7: access to community water supply for urban and rural populations and populations served by sewage systems. Definitions of other possible indicators are given, for example, in the publication of the United Nations Statistical Office (*24*) that has already been mentioned. Further outputs are discussed in the article "Community water supply and excreta disposal in developing countries", published by WHO (*27*).

Access to services can be measured by variables such as those given in Table 4.10, section 3. Data relating to health services are probably the most widely used (see, for example, columns 4 and 5 of Table 4.7).

Table 4.9. Comparison of indicators of concern in nutritional surveillance and in other indicator systems [a]

Subject/Indicator	(1) Nutritional surveillance	(2) United Nations	(3) Basic needs	(4) UNSO[b] social indicators	(5) UNSO[b] welfare measures	(6) World Bank[c]	(7) WHO
Population		+	+	+			
Wealth/assets	+			+	+		+
Housing	+	+	+			+	+
Production		+					+
Employment	+	+	+	+			
Income		+		+			+
Consumption	+	+	+	+			+
Nutritional status	+			+		+	+
Health	+	+	+	+			+
Mortality	+	+	+	+			+
Life expectancy		+	+	+			+
Health services	+	+	+	+		+	+
Environment:							
— water	+	+	+		+	+	+
— sanitation		+					+
Education		+	+	+	+	+	+

[a] Based on ref. 1, 23, 24, 25, and 52.
[b] United Nations Statistical Office.
[c] Living Standards Measurement Program.

Flow variables

Whether to include flow variables – and, if so, which to select – depends on the use to which the information is to be put and the resources available. Purchasing power (which can include subsistence consumption and takes prices into account) is more likely than overall food supply to be the crucial factor determining a household's food consumption and may therefore be given priority. Lower priority should be given to approaches aimed essentially at producing food balance-sheets for given areas, even should such balance-sheets be feasible, which they generally are not because of difficulties in monitoring amounts of food traded. A consequence of giving priority to purchasing power as a determinant of nutritional outcome is that many factors not immediately related to food itself may be of importance in nutritional surveillance. Thus the choice of indicators is not necessarily directed toward food supply and distribution. The collection of flow variables generally requires carefully designed sample surveys, whereas certain resource and outcome variables may be obtained from administrative sources. Where ongoing multipurpose sample survey systems are established, both flow and resource variables can be obtained from the same system.

Certain flow data that are quite widely available and are potentially useful for nutritional surveillance are briefly reviewed below.

Table 4.10. Status indicators [a]

1. Economic status (wealth)

A.   Physical reproducible assets
    (1)   Housing: type of construction
                  number of rooms
                  occupants per room
                  electrification
                  water supply (see 2.A)
    (2)   Consumer durables: culture-specific, e.g., ownership of bicycle, radio, livestock
    (3)   Equipment: e.g., farm tools, trade tools
    (4)   Savings
B.   Physical non-reproducible assets (natural resources), e.g.,
    (1)   Land-holding size
    (2)   Water sources for agriculture
C.   Intangible non-financial assets, e.g.,
    (1)   education – grade reached
                  – years of education
    (2)   Literacy

2. Environment

A.   Water supply
    (1)   Type of water source for domestic use
    (2)   Distance to water source (seasonal)
    (3)   Quantity of water available (seasonal)
    (4)   Quality of water available (seasonal)
B.   Excreta and waste disposal
    (1)   Type of toilet facility
    (2)   Type of garbage disposal
C.   Crowding – as 1.A(1)

3. Access to services

A.   Health services
B.   Agricultural extension
C.   Irrigation
D.   Credit
E.   Production inputs (seed, fertilizer, etc.)

[a] Based on ref. 24 and *Report of the Ad Hoc Committee on Guidelines for Monitoring and Evaluation of Rural Development as a Follow-up of WCAARD,* Rome, Food and Agriculture Organization of the United Nations, 1980 (mimeographed document).

Food balance sheets

This technique uses production and trade data, making adjustments for non-food use, storage, and processing losses, etc. by means of a "supply-utilization account", to give national estimates of energy and protein available for human consumption. Food balance sheets, produced domestically or prepared by FAO, (e.g., ref. *28*) are available for most countries. They usually go back two years or so, and time-series data can be obtained from them by year-to-year comparisons. At the national level, food balance-sheets have well-tried uses in overall planning. Moreover, the basic data that go into them are used for many other purposes, including trend analysis and the monitoring of production quantities and patterns, trade, utilization, losses, etc. For surveillance purposes, food balance sheet results are useful in giving an overall picture of trends in consumption patterns; however, they will only reflect changes in consumption requiring action at national level that are sufficiently important – such as the effects of drought – to be known from other sources. The production of food balance-sheets is not usually of high priority in nutritional surveillance programmes.

Agricultural production

Of potential interest for inclusion in long-term surveillance systems are data describing agricultural production levels retrospectively, disaggregated by the usual factors such as administrative area, ecology, farming pattern, etc. Early forecasts of agricultural production are more relevant to early warning and intervention programmes, as discussed in Chapter 6.

Although not often very accurate, data on crop production are widely available. They are derived from:

(a) estimates of areas planted and yields, based either on sample crop-cutting surveys or on estimates by agricultural extension workers;

(b) surveys of sample farms, in which both areas and yields are measured;

(c) for marketed production, records at buying-points, stocks held and distributed, etc.

These data are usually provided in aggregate form for the larger administrative areas, districts, provinces, etc. At this level, such information as may have been obtained at source – e.g., on types of farm, access to inputs – is not often used or passed on. Figures on such items are available, usually with a time lag of 1–2 years, in many countries. Although their accuracy is not high, they are of potential use in nutritional surveillance for monitoring food production trends and patterns by area. Production is mainly of interest in so far as it determines consumption. Changes in food production patterns will tend to be related to food consumption and nutrition when: (a) food production is the main source of cash income in the area; or (b) the farming in the area is primarily of a subsistence character.

A better indication of production, more closely related to consumption and nutritional status, has on occasions been obtained by combining food and non-food items to give estimates of the total value of agricultural production. An example from Kenya is shown in Table 4.11. Such data require the attribution of prices to different products and are of use in estimating incomes; they are usually derived from sample surveys. Time-series data would be particularly useful here. Suitable estimates could be derived from routine production statistics and used for regional comparisons and trend analyses. Data on modern sector agriculture for the major marketed crops are generally more easy to obtain and more accurate than data on traditional subsistence-oriented agriculture.

Table 4.11. Average value per holding of farm production and costs in Kenya, by province, excluding pastoral and large farm areas (in Kenyan shillings)[a]

	Central	Coast	Eastern	Nyanza	Rift Valley	Western	Total farm production
Farm production							
Crops sold to cooperatives[b]	510	117	512	592	380	61	428
Crops sold to local markets[c]	270	53	246	594	210	250	331
Net sales of cattle	218	154	299	161–	577	136	143
Net sales of other stock	122	99	134	10	260	42	88
Sales of milk	371	126	143	149	479	61	201
Total sales	1 491	549	1 334	1 184	1 906	550	1 192
Output used as seed	29	12	81	15	4	5	31
Output given to labour	19	17	21	13	26	16	18
Output fed to stock	101	24	13	12	55	15	35
Output consumed by household	1 530	670	1 667	1 047	1 686	896	1 297
Crop valuation change	20	110	115–	383	96	5	89
Livestock valuation change	52–	161–	513–	450	264	34	2–
Total production	3 138	1 221	2 488	3 104	4 063	1 521	2 659
Farm costs							
Total purchased crop inputs	271	31	202	137	391	96	185
Total livestock expenses	156	2	34	3	162	16	56
Total wages to labour	227	242	149	99	284	119	161
Total own produced inputs	149	53	115	40	85	36	84
Farm Repairs	217	64	77	35	28	69	92
Total farm costs	1 020	392	577	314	950	335	579
Farm operating surplus	2 120	828	1 911	2 789	3 086	1 186	2 081
Number of holdings	329 530	69 861	353 159	386 431	89 823	254 618	1 483 422

[a] Source: ref. 53, p. 66.
[b] Includes all direct sales to cooperatives and marketing boards.
[c] Includes sales to traders and board agents.

Data on livestock production present problems, particularly when traditional means of production are used. The sources of routine data in this area tend to be relatively unreliable and the possibilities for the widespread use of such data (without sample surveys) seem less promising.

Income, expenditure, and derived consumption data

Data on income and expenditure are usually derived from surveys of sample households. If data on nutritional status or food consumption have been collected in the same survey, then nutritional status can be analysed by income group and by proportion of total income allocated to food. An example from Costa Rica of such an output is given in Table 4.12. It has, however, seldom proved possible to link nutritional status and household budget data from separate surveys; efforts could be made to achieve better linkages in future, for example, by using overlapping samples.

Household budget surveys are probably the commonest source of information on income and expenditure. They usually cover expenditure on different items, including food commodities, and may or may not record quantities (as opposed to value), of food bought or purchase prices. The inclusion of quantities greatly enhances the utility of the survey for providing information on descriptive variables. If quantities (which may be in locally familiar units) are recorded, or if they can be calculated from expenditure and prices, then the energy and nutrient equivalents can be calculated from food tables (*29, 30*). To compute daily per capita intakes, both the demographic composition of each household and the period of time over which each item is consumed should ideally be known. In the aggregate, the rate of food purchase is sometimes taken to be equivalent to the rate of consumption. Demographic data are also desirable to allow calculated intakes to be compared with requirements.

Suitably treated, budget survey data may, on balance, be the best widely available source of information on food availability at the household level. Their validity needs to be checked by comparison with data on food consumption obtained by more accurate methods (e.g., by direct weighing, see below); these methods are, however, much more expensive and the results are accordingly less widely available than those based on household budget surveys. Several problems remain in interpreting the results, particularly if the data are highly disaggregated. For example, normal family consumption patterns may vary from week to week, as may individual energy consumption and expenditure; errors in the measurement of energy intake at the level of the individual units can be considerable, even though they may offset one another in the process of averaging (*31-33*).

Food consumption data

The direct weighing of food consumed can yield more accurate estimates of food intakes than those derived from household budget surveys. The crucial relationship between income and food consumption could only have been

Table 4.12. Distribution of children aged 0–5 years
in categories of weight-for-age according to monthly family
income level for the whole of Costa Rica [a]

Level of family income (colones)	Number of cases	Categories of weight-for-age			
		Overweight		Malnutrition	
			Normal	Grade I	Grades II & III
Less than 600	284	4.3	41.5	41.5	12.7
601– 800	246	6.1	38.6	42.7	12.6
801– 1 000	228	10.5	35.1	44.3	10.1
1 001– 1 500	757	8.1	38.5	43.5	9.9
1 501– 2 000	625	11.5	40.6	40.7	7.2
2 001– 2 500	362	11.6	47.1	31.1	10.2
2 501– 3 000	249	10.0	49.2	36.4	4.4
3 001– 4 000	289	13.5	49.0	28.1	9.4
4 001– 5 000	141	21.4	41.4	34.3	2.9
5 001– 6 000	108	24.1	47.2	25.9	2.8
6 001– 8 000	92	20.9	50.5	26.4	2.2
8 001–10 000	38	27.2	50.3	22.5	0.0
10 001 and more	24	30.0	49.1	20.9	0.0

[a] Source: ref. 54, p. 34.

Table 4.13. Energy intake and energy requirements
per person per day by income (Tunisia) [a]

	All	Income (dinars)									
		< 30	30– 60	60– 80	80– 100	100– 120	120– 160	160– 200	200– 300	300– 400	>400
Rural											
Intake	2474	1920	2168	2431	2437	2569	2702	2837	3065	3013	3126
Requirements	2132	2042	2117	2112	2122	2123	2140	2169	2221	2323	2240
Urban											
Intake	2228	1415	1809	1981	2200	2217	2302	2381	2569	2883	2899
Requirements	2199	2064	2074	2156	2202	2136	2169	2269	2310	2393	2436
Large cities											
Intake	2122	1077	1429	1829	1854	1913	2223	2219	2219	2518	2469
Requirements	2244	2086	2145	2161	2167	2277	2245	2190	2255	2335	2382

[a] Source: ref. 55.

demonstrated on the basis of such estimates. A good example is given in
Table 4.13: the probability of low consumption increases with decreasing
income. However, such data are probably not often needed and, in view of the
high cost and difficulty of food consumption surveys, are not regularly included
in surveillance systems.

Price data

Retail price indices are available in many developing countries, at least for major towns. These involve calculations based on standardized expenditure patterns (e.g., "food baskets"). In surveillance, the main uses of such data are for calculating changes in real income and estimating the extent to which changes in consumption are due to price changes. Estimates of the likely effects of price changes on consumption require values for price elasticities, which must be derived from household budget surveys, preferably repeated on several occasions, the price changes being recorded as well as expenditure/consumption.

In Costa Rica and El Salvador time-series data on food prices have been used and related to changes over a period of time in the minimum or real wages of different groups of labourers. The cost of a food-basket in Costa Rica has been expressed in terms of the hours of work needed in order to buy it, according to prevailing wages and food prices. The changes over a nine-year period in the hours of work needed in order to buy a food-basket are shown in Fig. 4.2.

The relationship of nutritional surveillance to price monitoring lies in the provision of nutritional information that may be of help in assessing the effects of price changes rather than data to guide price policy. Thus nutritional surveillance could conceivably have a special role, either in countries where the manipulation of food prices to improve consumption is a feature of national policy, or in those where there is concern about a deterioration in nutrition due to price increases (whether deliberate or not). In such cases, the main requirement will be a suitable comparison between outcome data and prices.

Formats for data outputs

The basic outputs from nutritional surveillance generally take the form of values for variables of interest classified by population group or area, a common example being data on prevalence of malnutrition by administrative area (e.g., district). These are usually presented in the form of one-way tabulations (e.g. prevalence of malnutrition by district) or two-way cross-tabulations (e.g., prevalence of malnutrition by district and family occupation, or relative prevalences of different degrees of malnutrition by district). The presentation is unavoidably two-dimensional – on a sheet of paper – and this imposes some constraints on output, at least to ensure that the results are comprehensible. Further analysis of the data normally requires more sophisticated techniques. By far the most common output therefore is the presentation of results by group. Whether the data are actually shown in the form of graphs, maps, histograms, or tables is generally a matter of presentation, not analysis.

The values in tabulated outputs are usually of three main types:

– the mean of a derived variable for the group concerned (e.g., mean weight-for-age);

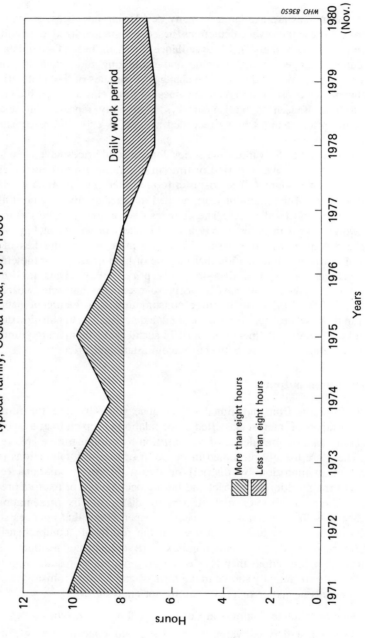

Fig. 4.2. Hours of work necessary per day to buy a food basket for a typical family, Costa Rica, 1971–1980

WHO 83650

– the proportion of the population below a cut-off point (e.g., for prevalence of malnutrition), or having a particular characteristic (e.g., for unprotected water supply);

– a composite index, such as a retail price index.

Composite indices have been explored in order to derive scores that describe, for example, level of living (see, for example, ref. *34*); these are not widely used at national level and will not be pursued further here. The relative merits of using means as opposed to proportions below cut-off points have been widely discussed elsewhere (*35*). Indicators that capture more of the overall characteristics of the distribution (e.g., Z-scores) have also been adopted in some cases (e.g., ref. *22*, p. 117). Prevalences of disease, recorded as sick/well, or mortality, are conceptually similar to proportions. Generally, proportions are more easily understood than means and hence more commonly used for presenting information.

The variables presented are often called "indicators". Indicators are variables themselves. The term often refers to ratios of other variables, such as proportions or prevalences. In the context of evaluation, indicators have been defined as "variables that help to measure changes" (*36*, p. 18). In nutritional surveillance, outcome variables are generally referred to as indicators, whether they are prevalences or proportions – which they most often are – or means, which are also used. For present purposes, "outcome variable" is synonymous with "indicator" or "outcome indicator". The expression has further connotations: it implies that the variable reflects some characteristic beyond its own precise meaning; prevalence of stunting in children may be taken to "indicate" level of nutrition in general; and this may indeed be valid. Too much significance should not be attached to the term "indicator", or to what the indicators used in this instance are "proxies" for. The indicators are used in a diagnostic way: a high prevalence of stunting; a high child mortality rate, a crowded insanitary environment, and poor housing, and so on present a picture that hardly needs more elaboration to be understood. This use of the term "indicator" is also similar to that adopted by, for example the World Bank (*37*, pp. 30-31).

For ease of comprehension, indicators should be presented so that changes in the same direction have a similar interpretation – for example, so that an increase means deterioration. A "high is bad" convention is usual in nutritional surveillance. This is obvious with prevalence of malnutrition or mortality rates. Housing could be assessed in terms of "percentage with improved housing" or "percentage with unimproved housing" (likewise for other facilities); terms like the latter ("percentage with unimproved housing") are used here for the sake of consistency with nutritional and mortality indicators. For intercountry comparisons, the alternative convention has been proposed (see Table 4.8) – e.g., "% of children with adequate birth weight". Provided the same convention is adopted within any one system, confusion can generally be avoided.

In the field of social indicators, the presentation of multiple indicators is usual. Examples were given in Table 4.7 of typical indicators of living conditions such as are frequently used for intercountry comparisons. Very much the same type of indicator series is useful for nutritional surveillance. Outputs of multiple indicators (not to be confused with composite indicators) are more than a presentational device. The outputs of nutritional surveillance systems describe and follow nutritional conditions in order to answer the questions given in Table 3.1. One convenient way of presenting data for this purpose is to provide a pattern of carefully chosen indicators that give a diagnostic picture of the situation.

An example of a standardized format is given in Table 4.14. The indicators can be either values at one time, or changes over time. Although the precise choice of indicators depends both on the local situation and the availability of data, the examples given are in fact widely applicable. Results should be reported both in terms of indicators for the whole group – irrespective of the group's size – and in the form of a proportion, e.g., percentage of malnourished subjects in the group.

Table 4.14. Example of format
for presenting an indicator series by group

Indicators	Group 1, 2 . . . n	Total
Total population in group		
% population in group		
Nutrition [a, b]		
% children < 80% Wt/Age		
% children < 90% Ht/Age		
% children < 80% Wt/Ht		
etc.		
No. children (or households with children) < 90% Ht/Age in group		
% total children of < 90% Ht/Age in this group		
Health		
% children with diarrhoea		
% children with fever		
% children born and died (per year)		
Calculated total child deaths/year		
% total child deaths in this group		
Socioeconomic/environmental		
% households with unimproved housing		
% households with no toilet		
% households with unprotected water supply		

[a] Wt/Age means weight-for-age; Ht/Age means height-for-age; Wt/Ht means weight-for-height.

[b] < 80% Wt/Age etc. means less than 80% of the standard used, e.g., the 50th centile by the standards of the National Center for Health Statistics (56).

Tabulations of a series of indicators show nutritional outcome and certain conditioning factors by *association,* not *causality,* and this must be taken into account in the interpretation of the data. Take the following hypothetical cross-sectional output:

Province A	Nutrition (% children <80% Wt/Age)	Infant mortality rate	Water supply (% not safe)
All farmers	30	50	60
Modern sector	25	30	40
Traditional sector	35	70	80

It would not be valid to conclude from these data that the high prevalence of malnutrition and the high infant mortality rate among families of farmers in the traditional sector were due to the lack of a safe water supply; it would be reasonable, however, to decide that the malnutrition and high infant mortality were priority social problems and to investigate whether measures to improve the water supply were likely to prove effective as part of a programme aimed at this group, and, if so, what aspects of the water supply should be dealt with. Firm conclusions on water supply cannot come from an output such as this, but require more detailed analysis with the aim of getting closer to the causes of the situation. They may also require further small-scale studies. Strictly speaking, causes are impossible to establish with epidemiological data such as these, and experimental interventions are needed for the purpose. However, a rigidly logical approach may not always be feasible or even necessary.

The presentation of data as a series of indicators serves several purposes that have to be reconciled. The first purpose is to present more relevant information at a glance; another is to lead to some synthesis of the information without, at that stage, needing to use sophisticated analytical techniques. The objectives of summarization, disaggregation, and synthesis pull in different directions, and need to be balanced. The output needs to be as simple as possible, while capturing the meaning of the results.

An indicator series will show that certain values move in the same direction, and others not, which complicates interpretation; this applies between groups at one time, or between different times for the same group. It is evident that other knowledge about the specific situation being assessed will be needed. As a rule of thumb, it seems not unreasonable to propose the following:

– when indicators correspond (move in the same direction between groups or over time), general features of the situation as well as specific problems are being traced, and both general and specific solutions can be considered;

– when indicators do not correspond, specific problems are being identified for which specific solutions may be required.

Testing significance of results

The levels of the outcome indicators relate both to differences between groups and to changes over time. Estimates are necessary to see whether large differences are likely to be significant. A few important points need to be borne in mind here.

With many of the results from nutritional surveillance, conventional statistical tests of significance apply only approximately because the sample is not random and the distribution of values not normal. Furthermore, the conventional levels of significance may sometimes be relaxed – for planning and management decisions, 95% certainty is often impossible, and a three-to-one chance, say, would be satisfactory. However, two of the most common procedures used in statistics meet many of the requirements for assessing the significance of nutritional surveillance results. These are the chi-square test applied to prevalences or proportions; and, in the consideration of means, the analysis of variance (equivalent to a t-test when applied to two groups). Detailed discussion of these procedures is beyond the scope of this book, but descriptions of them are available in standard texts (e.g., ref. *38*).

Combining of indicators

A series of indicators can give more information than single indicators presented separately. An example is provided by Table 4.15, which illustrates the correspondence between a series of indicators, albeit employing cross-sectional data. Here the presentation broadly quantifies the need of the more isolated communities – in terms of malnutrition, child mortality, morbidity, and housing – more effectively than any one of these indicators separately would have done. It is also important to show relative numbers of households affected, as well as proportions or prevalences. This corresponds to the standardized format shown in Table 4.14. The use of such indicator series is only beginning in nutritional surveillance, and in fact it has so far been confined to Costa Rica. Other examples have therefore been drawn up from existing data to illustrate their use.

One of the most effective outputs of the SIN in Costa Rica was to present a series of indicators by administrative area, as shown in Table 4.16. This was based on a survey of schoolchildren's heights, together with data from earlier censuses of population and housing. The impact of this presentation was much greater than would have been possible by the use of any of the single indicators previously used. In fact it was not necessary to go further in examining correlations. This illustrates the *diagnostic* use of data from various sources. A later step will obviously be to look at changes over time in the individual indicators.

A first step in presenting a series of indicators is to put together nutritional and health outcome indicators. This can be done cross-sectionally and in time-series fashion. Certain results from the Central American countries covered by the Institute of Nutrition of Central America and Panama (INCAP) can be treated in this way as an illustration. Table 4.17 shows nutritional status, mortality rates, and estimates of food availability for Costa Rica, El Salvador, and Guatemala for 1965–78. Certain socioeconomic indicators can be added, giving

Table 4.15. Example of series of indicators by group,
from survey in Haiti [a]

Indicator	Time to reach town (administrative centre) in minutes				Total
	0–50	50–100	100–200	200	
Number of households in sample	41	72	106	42	261
Number of children in sample	67	120	174	69	430
Population % in group	15.7	27.6	40.6	15.7	100
Number of households in group	3140	5520	8130	3140	19 930
Nutrition [b]: %<90% Ht/Age	34.3	35.0	54.0	62.3	47.0
%<80% Wt/Age	32.8	49.2	57.5	53.6	50.7
% total malnourished in group	10.2	26.8	46.1	16.6	100
Mortality: % children born and died	13.4	13.1	17.2	22.5	16.5
Morbidity: % sick in preceding week	44.8	50.8	57.5	63.8	54.7
Wealth: % unimproved housing	19.5	26.4	35.8	33.3	30.3

[a] Source: ref. 57.
[b] Ht/Age = height-for-age; Wt/Age = weight-for-age.

Table 4.18. The use of absolute numbers as well as rates gives a view of the relative sizes of nutrition/health problems. For example, 62% of all infant deaths in the three countries were in Guatemala. If these indicators were in fact for three regions within a country, they would have important implications for the regional allocation of resources, both generally for economic development and specifically for social services. These results are now easier to interpret in relation to the questions in Table 3.1. The health and nutrition situation clearly improved over the years in all three countries, but the trend was not the same in each of them. Costa Rica and El Salvador showed similar declines in the prevalence of second- and third-degree malnutrition (0.41%–0.45% per year), which was about twice the rate for Guatemala; most of the improvement in Costa Rica was in the years 1975–78. The infant mortality rate declined more rapidly in Costa Rica than in the other two countries, the rates of decline in Guatemala and El Salvador being somewhat less than the regional average. These results indicate that Guatemala not only remains worst off from the standpoint of nutrition and infant mortality, but is showing the slowest rate of improvement in nutrition. The results as they stand do not identify the specific measures needed beyond showing that Guatemala is relatively poorly covered by health services. The next step would be to break down the cross-sectional and time-series data by socioeconomic group.

A second example, from a survey in Egypt, illustrates the use of existing cross-sectional survey data to give a series of indicators. This is presented in Table 4.19, which is based on several tables in the survey report (22). Chronic

Table 4.16. Social profile of the 10 cantons with highest and lowest levels of height retardation in children attending first grade of primary school. Height census of 1979 and population and housing census of 1973, Costa Rica [a]

Level of height retardation and canton	Percentage of children with following characteristics:				
	Height retardation [b]	Illiteracy	Poor dwelling	Dwellings without latrines	Dwellings without running water
High height retardation					
Coto Brus	24.6(1 045)	17.9	20.2	39.2	78.2
Los Chiles	23.1(485)	34.8	15.8	53.3	88.8
Buenos Aires	23.0(824)	23.4	29.2	51.6	84.2
Aserrí	22.8(758)	12.6	17.4	15.8	11.8
Pocosí	22.1(1 137)	14.7	15.3	18.9	61.8
Turrubares	21.7(184)	30.1	17.4	37.4	45.0
Guatuso	21.6(259)	28.6	16.1	44.0	87.2
Guácimo	21.3(286)	17.5	14.9	21.3	54.7
Tarruzú	21.2(212)	15.7	18.4	18.0	17.8
Golfito	21.0(891)	16.7	11.8	23.9	38.0
Low height retardation					
Tibás	7.0(884)	3.7	10.2	0.7	1.0
Moravia	6.9(435)	3.1	7.8	1.9	5.4
Alfaro Ruiz	6.8(133)	6.8	5.8	2.4	12.2
Montes de Oca	6.4(466)	3.0	8.2	0.8	1.7
Barva	6.4(282)	6.2	11.2	1.8	1.8
Central San José	6.3(4 193)	3.5	10.4	0.4	0.9
Atenas	5.7(297)	10.5	15.3	7.4	14.8
Goicochea	5.3(1 183)	3.7	9.2	0.7	1.5
Palmares	4.9(268)	6.2	8.4	7.1	8.0
Belén	4.4(203)	5.3	5.9	3.6	1.9

[a] Source: ref. 58.
[b] In parenthesis the number of children evaluated by canton in height census of 1979.

child malnutrition is seen to be concentrated in the rural areas and large villages, which are much more poorly served with water supplies and have higher illiteracy rates. Their households are characterized by dependence on small-holder farming, farm labour, and share-cropping. Indeed, the correspondence between dependence on farm labour, by zone and chronic malnutrition is surprisingly close. Malnutrition is probably concentrated in the households of small farmers, farm labourers, etc., in the rural areas, and these families probably do not have piped water or literate heads-of-household. Further tabulations by such categories as occupational groups within zones, access to water, etc., would demonstrate such factors. Multivariate analyses to examine the relative influence of different factors would give some insight into possible causal relationships and indicate specific measures to be taken.

Table 4.17. Example of synthesis of results to give a series of indicators, from data on Central American countries, 1965-1978 [a]

Indicator	Costa Rica			El Salvador		Guatemala		
	1966	1975	1978	1965	1976	1965	1976	1977
Nutritional status (NS):								
% grades II and III by Wt/Age	13.5	12.3	8.6	27.5	22.6	33.6	34.6	30.5
Infant mortality rate (IMR)	65.1	37.9	24.0	70.6	58.1 (1975)	92.6	76.3	
Child mortality rate	6.3	2.2		15.0	6.4	33.5	21.0	
Change per year absolute NS		0.41			0.45		0.26	
Change per year absolute IMR		3.4			1.3		1.5	
Change per year relative to 1965/6 NS		3.0			1.6		0.8	
Change per year relative to 1965/6 IMR		5.3			1.8		1.6	

[a] Source: ref. 25 and 28.

Table 4.18. Series of selected indicators for Costa Rica, El Salvador, and Guatemala: cross-sectional presentation [a]

Indicator	Costa Rica	El Salvador	Guatemala	Total
Total population ($\times 10^3$)	1572	3555	5160	10 287
% population in group	17.7	33.6	48.7	100
Total child population, 0–5 years ($\times 10^3$)	374	711	1032	2117
Nutritional status:				
% grades II and III by Wt/Age	12.3 ('75)	22.6 ('76)	34.6 ('76)	
Total no. grades II and III by Wt/Age	46	161	357	564
% total grades II and III by Wt/Age	8.2	28.5	63.3	100
Infant mortality rate	37.9	58.1 ('75)	76.3	
Child mortality rate	2.2	6.4	21.0	
Calculated total infant deaths/year [b]	1 987	8 055	16 142	26 184
% total infant deaths	7.6	30.7	61.6	
Population per physician (1976)	1 550	3 460	2 500	
% no access to safe water	23	47	60	
% illiterate	11	42	53	
Income share, upper 60%	85	92.5	78	

[a] Source: ref. 25 and 59.
[b] From birth rate data, not shown.

Table 4.19. Indicator series for Egypt taken from various survey tables of the Centers for Disease Control [a]

Indicator	Lower rural	Upper rural	Large villages	Small towns	Small cities	Total	Cairo-Gaza	Alexandria
Population in group ($\times 10^3$)	8 539	6 433	5 516	2 762	4 492	27 742	1 334	552
% population in group	30.8	23.2	19.9	10.0	16.2	100		
% children Wt/Ht<85%	2.4	2.9	1.9	2.5	1.3	2.3	3.5	0.5
% children Wt/Age<75%	8.4	12.9	9.7	6.7	3.8	8.8	9.3	4.8
% children Ht/Age<90%	21.8	27.5	24.3	14.8	10.6	21.2	19.0	15.7
% children Hb < 9.5 S/100 ml	14.9	16.5	11.9	8.3	3.3	12.2	5.6	11.8
Total no. stunted children ($\times 10^3$)	1 862	1 769	1 340	408	476	5 855		
% total stunted children	31.8	30.2	22.9	7.0	8.1	100		
% children with recent diarrhoea	8.7	10.8	10.0	7.8	9.4	9.5	14.0	20.6
% children with recent fever	17.3	15.0	16.6	11.5	15.3	15.7	17.3	30.6
% households without piped water or well water	87.8	82.8	73.1	51.3	20.5	—	50.3	50.3
% households with illiterate father	54.0	68.1	58.2	42.9	26.8	52.4	48.5	55.4
% households with small farmers, labourers, etc.	80.0	86.8	80.2	55.7	45.2	73.2	62.3	75.0
% households with labourers	23.1	32.8	29.6	8.8	2.3	21.6	12.2	7.6

[a] Source: Compiled from several tables in ref. 22.

Data Sources

Data for nutritional surveillance are obtained largely from existing sources, i.e., administrative sources or surveys; the latter are often carried out for a number of different purposes. Occasionally, special collections of data may be undertaken to investigate particular problems. The types of data obtainable from different sources are shown in Table 4.20. The actual use of these data sources in selected surveillance systems is shown in Table 4.21. Data are almost always drawn from the health system; local government sources are also common. The use of data from schools, while promising, has yet to be more widely developed. Household surveys are available in several countries; in Kenya they form the major source of data, and in Costa Rica and Sri Lanka they are widely used to supplement existing data. This section reviews the principles governing the identification and use of sources of data for nutritional surveillance, drawing as before on certain examples from existing systems.

Table 4.20. Types of data from existing sources
used in nutritional surveillance systems

Source	Variables	
	Actual	Potential
Clinics (health personnel)	Weight, height, age Disease prevalence Immunization record Birth weights By location	Occupation, etc. Distance from clinic of home
Schools	Weight, height, age By location	Occupation, etc. Distance of home from school
Administrative records	Births Child mortality rates	Occupation, etc. Birth weights
Retail price reporting	Market prices of food By location	Food shortages, availability
Census - demographic, housing, agricultural	Demographic, socioeconomic, agricultural, environmental variables	
Household surveys	Socioeconomic variables	Weight, height, age
Agricultural reports	Crop production (yields, areas)	Agricultural resources
Village reports	Services, infrastructure, health environment, distance data	
Ministry of labour – labour force surveys	Minimum wage rates Actual wage rates	
Non-specific sources (i.e., any of the above)		Services, infrastructure, health environment, distance data

Administrative data

Sources of administrative data depend on existing services, usually government ones. They do not therefore usually cover a predefined sample of
individuals, households, or sites. Administrative sources are particularly useful
for obtaining data on levels of resources and outcome; data on outcome tend to
be more readily available than data on resources. Moreover, administrative data
tend to be more widely available and may be more disaggregated (e.g., they may
be available for specific villages) than sample survey data.

The selection of sources depends on balancing data requirements against
potential availability. The chain of thought might be as follows: outcome
indicators are needed; infant and child mortality would be ideal. Can reliable
data be obtained at reasonable cost, since the completeness of registration of

Table 4.21. Data sources used in selected
nutritional surveillance systems

	Clinics/ health workers	Schools	Local govt. admin. records	Census	Agric. reports	Community weighing	Retail price reporting	Village surveys	Household surveys
Chile	+		+	+					
Colombia	+		+		+		+		
Costa Rica	+	+	+	+			+	+	+
El Salvador	+		+	+			+		
Kenya									+
Philippines		+				+			
Sri Lanka	+								+

births and infant deaths is known to vary? Or would it be better to use data on children at school entry, which are already being widely collected in schools, but not transmitted at present? What size should the sample of schools be, and how much would the operation cost? In the long term, should the major effort go into improving vital registration through local government?

Obviously, it is easier to set up the data collection system where the data are being gathered anyway, even if they are not centralized or otherwise reported on. This is true in the case of health, school, local government, and agricultural records, and could also be applicable to such potential sources as reports on prices, minimum wages, etc. It is clear that only limited amounts of information can be requested from the relevant services, particularly if collecting such information is not part of the routine duties of the staff. On the other hand, it may be possible to modify data that are already being collected so that they are more useful for nutritional surveillance: this was the case, for example, with socioeconomic information collected by Costa Rican health agents. Four situations are possible:

(a) Data are being collected peripherally and transmitted to central points (e.g., ministries of agriculture or health), but are not being interpreted and utilized for surveillance purposes. This is commonly the case – for instance, with health/nutrition data in El Salvador before 1977 (39).

(b) Data exist but are not being transmitted. This was the case with anthropometric data from the health sector in Costa Rica and probably applies to anthropometric school data from a number of countries, particularly in Latin America where school enrolment is high. In this situation, the requirements are:

— administrative arrangements for capturing the data, provision of forms, agreement on procedures, etc.;

— the training or retraining of personnel in measurement techniques and motivation;

— the possible provision of additional personnel;
— the provision, maintenance, and standardization of equipment;
— quality control of the data, using the existing supervisory structure as far as possible.

In deciding on the possible operation of a surveillance system, the feasibility of meeting these requirements will be one factor to be considered.

(c) Personnel are available who could in principle collect data but are not doing so at present. The collection of data from schools is an example of this. In this case, it becomes necessary for those initiating surveillance to reach agreement with the relevant authorities, and then to consider requirements similar to those in (b) above.

(d) There is no data collection at present and personnel would have to be hired specifically for the routine collection of data. This is likely to be a serious constraint, and it is unlikely that starting from scratch would be justifiable exclusively for purposes of surveillance. It might, however, be justified if there were other uses for the data, e.g., for individual screening.

Data gathered from routine services, such as clinics, are of unknown validity with respect to the population as a whole, and due account must be taken of this constraint when considering the use of administrative sources of data. Two questions should be looked into at the outset. First, representative sample surveys may be needed to gain information on the extent to which routine data and changes deduced from them in fact reflect the situation in the population covered. Secondly, the possibility of collecting a few items of additional information in order to define the population covered should be investigated. If certain characteristics of the population and of those attending the clinic are noted and tested for their stability, the changes observed in the characteristics of those attending the clinic may still permit useful inferences to be made, albeit not in a statistical sense, about changes in the situation of the population. This is possible if baseline linkages between the characteristics of the population and the non-random sample are found through representative sample surveys and by collecting a few items of additional information in order to define the population covered. For example, changes in the outreach of health services might be monitored by means of information on occupation and location in terms of distance from the clinic. In general, such data may be more reliable for detecting changes, over time in one location (e.g., a clinic) than for comparing different locations at one point in time.

The use of individual administrative sources of data is now discussed in more detail.

Health

There are two ways in which data can be derived from the health system. First, arrangements may be made for transmission to a central analytical unit of some or all of the following data on children:

— weights, heights and ages
— immunizations
— birth weights
— diagnosed illnesses.

The data are usually obtained on all children presenting at clinics; the clinics themselves are selected from all the health facilities in the area. This method is used, for example, in Colombia and El Salvador. The analysis can be based on a sampling of records and should be carried out at roughly monthly intervals. Secondly, health agents can be used to acquire information from home visits scheduled as part of their duties; this can include socioeconomic information as well as data on health and nutritional status, as in Costa Rica.

The important decision has always to be made whether all cases will be reported, or whether a sample will be taken. In the former eventuality, records can be sampled at a later stage. In principle, it is better to draw a sample from a larger number of data sources (e.g., clinics), than to process the records of all the cases from a smaller number of sources. Some form of selection is needed, and clearly it is more economical to record only those data that will be used. This means that a system of sampling should be established in clinics used as data sources.

The procedure that has been adopted to draw upon data from the health system, following discussion and agreement with the health authorities, has involved:

— reviews and discussions of the existing reporting system;
— the provision of forms (which may even be simplified versions of previous forms) for reporting data from clinics or household visits (these can cover identification, anthropometric measurements, diagnosed illnesses and immunization, or provide for reports of birth weights);
— the training of health supervisors to instruct health personnel in measurement and interview techniques;
— the provision of equipment (scales, height boards) if not already available;
— arrangements for transmission of data;
— procedures for controlling data quality.

The time required for extending this system to clinics, where the data were already being collected, was a matter of months in most cases (e.g., Colombia, Costa Rica, El Salvador); the most usual bottleneck was data analysis, compounded by inadequate sampling of clinics or of records.

Education

Teachers can contribute data to surveillance systems by measuring the heights and sometimes the weights of children on school entry. Community weighing programmes for preschool children (as in the Philippines, for example) are also assisted by teachers and are discussed separately below.

The recording of anthropometric information on children at school entry is particularly valuable for the long-term monitoring of nutrition. Since it applies only to children attending school, it may in some cultures exclude the more deprived members of the community. Additional information can be gained on the socioeconomic status of the children measured, e.g., on parents' occupations. The requirements for obtaining anthropometric information on school-children include:

– agreement with the education authorities and the cooperation of the teachers concerned;

– technical documentation, training, reporting forms, equipment.

To give an example of this process, in Costa Rica a survey of the nutritional status of schoolchildren in 1979 took 12 months from the initial contacts with the Ministry of Education until the reports giving the main findings became available. Five months were necessary for contacts with the Ministry of Education, the preparation of instructions for the teachers, validation exercises, the establishment of quality control systems, the design of the measuring instrument, and the definition of the data flow mechanism. The actual data collection took place in a single week and demanded two hours of the time of each first-grade teacher. Data flow, checking of forms for gross errors, and the processing, analysis, and preparation of reports took seven months. However, preparations for a second survey, conducted in June 1981, started in May of that year and reports were available by November.

The idea of organizing the collection by teachers of data on the community is particularly attractive in that the education system (like health, agriculture, and local government) tends to be spread throughout the country and, moreover, to be staffed with relatively well-educated people. A fund of goodwill often exists that can be fruitfully tapped – or wastefully exploited. It is especially important, therefore, to ensure that the additional work the teachers are asked to carry out, which will necessarily lie outside their main duties, is put to good use. If there is a possibility of cooperation by teachers in obtaining information on the community at large for purposes of nutrional surveillance, it is more important than ever that the uses to which the data will be put should be clearly thought out and discussed with those involved.

Agriculture

Only minor use has been made so far of information from agricultural reports in nutritional surveillance. There may be several reasons for this. First, the potential uses of the data have been insufficiently specified: for development planning such data would be used to follow changes and trends in production by area on a year-to-year (or season-to-season) basis, rather than to give early warning of crop failure. In agricultural communities, these changes would reflect changes in real income and would be expected to have a bearing on nutritional outcome. Secondly, there are administrative and intersectoral reasons why the data have not been used: administrative arrangements for capturing them at the needed level of disaggregation may have been difficult. Thirdly, the data are known to be of questionable reliability, both from the standpoint of accuracy (since guesswork is often involved) and from that of systematic reporting.

These constraints could be overcome if the use of agricultural reports were seen to be worth while. Requirements for developing the system would be somewhat analogous to those for developing health reporting:

– agreement with agricultural services on reporting procedures;
– technical documentation on procedures, provision of or modification to forms;
– the training or retraining of personnel;
– quality control of the data.

Local government administration

Two types of information from local government administrations are of particular interest: registration of births and deaths, and data applying to villages or areas on infrastructure, services, etc.

Local administrative records have been used to extract data on infant and child mortality rates. These vital statistics are recorded primarily for legal reasons. Birth certificates serve as proof of identity and are required for various purposes throughout life. Death certificates are proof of death of an individual, needed for probates, burial permits, etc. Hence there are important reasons for the recording of such information. Birth and death registers contain information that is potentially useful for nutritional surveillance, for example, causes of death listed by age, sex and residence. As legal documents, birth and death certificates may be kept by the civil service or various other organizations rather than the health sector. Some examples follow. In rural India, the registration of births and deaths is the responsibility of the local government, the revenue service, the police agency, and/or the health agency (*40*, p. 13). In Honduras, volunteer "health guardians" in villages report births and deaths to the secretaries of their respective municipalities (*16*, p. 6). The Filipino registrar is a local finance officer, a city health officer, or somebody appointed by the municipality (*16*, p. 153). In rural Thailand, the local village headman reports through the commune headman to the district officer (*16*, p. 153). In many cases, however, there is little training or supervision of the registrars and hence the accuracy of the reporting may be suspect. Indeed, the vital registration statistics of many developing countries are known to be rather incomplete. In 1973, an estimated 28-35% of the world's population had reliable data on live births; in Africa the proportion was 2-17%, and in Asia it was 7% (*41*, p. 10). However, many birth and death certificates also record such data as occupation, as well as location, and thus, if coverage were reasonable, could be a useful source of information.

Local government administrations can also help nutritional surveillance efforts by collecting more general information on villages. Certain information is potentially relatively easy to obtain at village level, if the administrative structure to report on it can be set up. This mainly applies to indicators such as:

- infrastructure (roads, community buildings);
- physical services such as water and electricity supply;
- access to health and education services;
- the agricultural pattern.

Such data can be used either as measures of level of development having implications for nutritional outcome, or as factors defining socioeconomic groups when linked with nutritional outcome data. This linkage can be performed by combining data from different sources at the level of the village.

The Village Classification Scheme in Malaysia is one example of a system that obtains this type of village-level data. Under this scheme, which covers approximately 4000 villages in Peninsular Malaysia, data have been collected by village in five broad areas: the basic administrative agricultural system; physical characteristics and services; economic development; land use and ownership; social development. Certain states in India have similar arrangements. As yet, such data have not been combined with nutritional data, but this could be done. The Costa Rican health system has data at the village level which include in aggregated form family/individual records, together with village characteristics, resources, and distances to cities or services. Since such data would be relatively cheap to collect, the investigation of their potential availability should be given some priority when nutritional surveillance systems are being set up.

The development of such a system would require inputs similar to those for other administrative sources of data:

- agreement with local authorities and agency personnel;
- the provision of technical documentation and forms;
- training;
- arrangements for data transmission;
- quality control of the data.

Census data

Although available only at long intervals – usually ten years – census data are useful for a number of purposes in nutritional surveillance. In particular, the censuses often provide the only data of wide coverage that can be highly disaggregated. Moreover, they are usually available in published form, though access to unpublished items is sometimes needed in order to have a sufficient degree of disaggregation. The uses of census data are as follows. First, they provide supplementary outcome indicators, which can usefully be added to nutritional or health data. For example, in Costa Rica, data on literacy and housing have been taken from census material; in Kenya, child mortality rates by district were derived from the census of 1979, and analysed by mother's educational level (51). Secondly, census data include numbers of individuals or households within relevant geographical or socioeconomic groupings; they can therefore be used to quantify the extent of nutritional problems identified from other sources. Thirdly, census data have been used for the extrapolation of nutritional data by means of statistical methods, based on associations between census variables and nutritional indicators: this was done, for example, in the Philippines to give estimates of prevalences of malnutrition by municipality.[1]

Community weighing programme

Nationwide infant- and child-weighing programmes exist in at least two countries, Indonesia and the Philippines. In the Philippines, the programme – called Operation Timbang – has been in operation since 1974 and originally aimed at yearly weighing of all children under the age of 5. This was done in each *barangay* (village), usually by schoolteachers. The programme has expanded to include the regular half-yearly weighing of preschool children and the quarterly weighing of children known to suffer from third-degree malnutrition. The weighing is increasingly being carried out by trained *barangay* nutrition and health scholars who at present cover more than 10% of the *barangays* in the country. The information collected (weight-for-age) is moved upward through health system channels to the National Nutrition Council and is available at the national, regional, provincial, and local levels for the setting of programme targets. The programme aims at 100% coverage of all children under 5, and no sampling is done. The present coverage is approximately 30%. The data, as collected at present, are probably most useful for setting targets at the local (municipal) level. Clear comparisons between regions are hindered by errors of measurement and reporting and by the fact that the incomplete coverage may systematically bias the data. For example, the mean prevalence of second- plus third-degree malnutrition according to the weighing programme is about 30%; according to representative sample surveys, it is about 22% (*42, 43*).

In Indonesia, a weighing programme was instituted in 1977 as part of the Family Nutrition Improvement Programme. Children under 5 years of age are weighed monthly by trained, local volunteers. Reporting is done through the nearest health centre, the data being finally aggregated at the national level. The collection, compilation, and display of the information are soon to be included in a national surveillance system. The coverage at present is around 80%. One constraint at present is that the huge masses of data being generated by the monthly weighings cannot be managed until the nutrition surveillance system is operable.

It is doubtful whether such community weighing programmes would be justifiable for purposes of nutritional surveillance alone. However, when such

---

[1] Philippines. NNC/Cornell. *Philippine Nutrition surveillance project.* Manila, NNC (with Cornell Nutritional Surveillance Program, Ithaca, NY), 1981.

programmes are instituted for individual screening and follow-up, they may prove a useful source of data. Record sampling for surveillance purposes may be indicated. Since data collection (and local analysis) capacity is limited, the trade-offs between frequency, coverage, and types of measurement need to be assessed for surveillance purposes. Less frequent collections of data (say, every year or every two years) with greater coverage, or deliberate sampling, would often provide useful information; similarly, the addition of a few more variables, such as socioeconomic status, would often greatly enhance the utility of the data. When the purpose is primarily screening, then the deciding factor is the capacity for intervention.

Household sample surveys

The use of household surveys to obtain data for nutritional surveillance depends largely on the pre-existence of suitable survey activities. The experience of the last few years is that very few survey systems dealing primarily with nutrition have been set up. This is probably due, quite simply, to the fact that surveys are expensive and are funded on a continuing basis only for data regarded as indispensable for government planning. Repetitions of isolated surveys can provide information potentially useful for nutritional surveillance (22).[1]

On the other hand, continuing or regular sample survey systems are becoming more common in developing countries. The system in Kenya is a good example, but not unique, except in including nutrition. Quite a number of countries have – or are developing – similar survey systems; these do not at present include nutrition measurements, but potentially could do so. Almost every country in the world has carried out some form of household survey in the past few years (see ref. 44, pp. 148-150).[2] An increasing trend at present is to develop surveys into ongoing systems. Certain of these surveys concentrate on specific themes (e.g., employment, literacy) year by year; others are multipurpose, introducing modules on specific topics as required. International support to household surveys is becoming available through the United Nations Household Survey Capability Programme (45).

A number of household surveys that were carried out on a "once-only" basis have provided nutritional data as a spin-off. Household budget surveys can be particularly useful, but often need some modifications. The following relatively low-cost additions to household budget surveys could therefore substantially extend their value for nutritional surveillance:

---

[1] See also: EGYPT. THE NUTRITION INSTITUTE. *Arab Republic of Egypt Nutrition Status Survey II*. Washington, DC. USAID, 1980 (mineographed document).

[2] See also: INTER-AMERICAN STATISTICAL INSTITUTE. *Bases for consideration of an Inter-American Household Survey Program (PIDEH)*. Washington, DC, IASI, 1980 (mineographed document 7610a-7/25/80-100).

— routine records of quantities of food purchased;
— records of the time in which the food is consumed and the prices paid for it (these can be obtained when collecting expenditure data);
— a better description of the demographic characteristics of the household;
— a calculation of the quantities of food available to the household, per head or consumption unit, in a given period (a day, 3 days, a week).

Regular or ongoing household surveys offer particular opportunities for developing nutritional surveillance. They could furnish indicators of food expenditure and availability from the data regularly collected, as well as offering the possibility of including a nutrition module (see next section).

Most household surveys organized by government departments to obtain general socioeconomic and/or agricultural data draw a sample from the population of the country as a whole, from large administrative areas within the country, or specifically from urban or rural sectors. The selection of the sample is usually done in two or more stages, beginning with clusters and then selecting households within the clusters. The sample is commonly stratified, i.e., clusters are selected within strata defined, for example, by area; data on characteristics pertaining to strata are then aggregated to the level of the population using the information that must be available on the size of each stratum. The sample size (which should be decided not as a proportion of the population, but from a consideration of the conclusions sought and the precision required) is usually within the range 1000–50 000 households, typical values being around 2000–10 000.

Data are collected, mainly by interview, in sample households. Material measurements can include size of land-holdings (total or cultivated), yields, etc. In certain food consumption surveys, weights of food either before cooking or as prepared are measured, often on repeated visits. Questionnaires may run to many pages and take two or more hours to administer, although it is commonly held that a questionnaire should not take more than one hour to complete. For certain types of data, repeated visits are often used: e.g., on several consecutive days for food consumption, every week or month for expenditure or income, and/or seasonally. The survey structure established to obtain these data involves teams of enumerators and supervisors. These must be trained for a few weeks at the beginning of the survey and retrained at intervals for long surveys, or when the questionnaire changes. A substantial administrative and logistical effort is needed to support these teams in the field.

Methods for household surveys are well documented in the literature, (see, for example, ref. *21, 45, 46*). The usefulness of these surveys in obtaining nutrition data depends partly on solving some of the general problems experienced with household surveys. These include inadequate questionnaire design, insufficient training of enumerators, and failure of logistical and administrative back-up. Success depends mainly on the adequate application of known methods and on the effective administration of established procedures.

Obtaining nutritional data from household surveys: use of a nutrition module

The use of existing or projected household surveys for obtaining data for nutritional surveillance requires:

– the regular inclusion of nutrition measurements in survey systems as a "nutrition module"; and/or

– the interpretation of data from the surveys in terms of nutrition, which itself may require the inclusion of a limited number of additional variables in the basic survey questionnaire. Considerations to be taken into account in deciding whether and how to include nutrition variables are discussed below.

The inclusion of a nutrition module within an ongoing survey system means that the survey capacity will be used for a limited period of time (e.g., one month) to collect data specifically on nutrition. Steps must therefore be taken to design a questionnaire, train enumerators, provide equipment, and arrange for supervision of the measurements and interviews. The module normally covers the entire sample.

It has been shown in Kenya that it is quite feasible to include a nutrition module in a general purpose survey system. The questionnaire used is given in Table 4.22. The criteria for this approach are fairly obvious: the existence of a suitable survey system into which a nutrition module can be introduced; the capacity of the system operate the module successfully; a need for the data; and the capacity to analyse and interpret the data. These criteria are discussed below.

An indispensable feature of surveys in which a nutrition module can suitably be included is that the data should be collected in sample *households*. They should be conducted by means of a questionnaire administered to members of the household (preferably including the wife or mother) by enumerators who can also take the children's measurements (if necessary, an additional enumerator may be employed for this purpose). In general, household budget or demographic surveys are suitable for the inclusion of a nutrition module, agricultural surveys or censuses probably less so, and physical surveys (e.g., of natural resources) obviously not.

The capacity of the enumerators, supervisors, and logistical support staff to handle the appropriate techniques and control the quality of the data needs to be assessed, but the difficulties involved, though substantial, should not be overestimated. In Kenya, a three-day training course for enumerators was found to be adequate, and provision of transport and maintenance of equipment did not pose overwhelming problems. Nevertheless, to overburden the survey – in terms of enumerator training, interview time, transport arrangements, etc. – would put the reliability of the data collection process at risk and could even lead to its breakdown. There is clearly a trade-off between including a nutrition module and collecting alternative data; a certain priority has to be given to nutrition if it is to find a place in the survey. This priority depends partly on the usefulness of the additional data as perceived by those responsible for the survey.

Table 4.22. Example of questionnaire for nutrition module in household survey [a]

Target Population: All children in the sample households between 1 year (i.e., 12 months) and 4 years (i.e., 48 months) of age.

CODE [b]

1	2	3	4	5	6	7	8

CARD NO.

9	0
9	10

PROVINCE _____ DISTRICT _____

LOCATION _____ DATE _____

Name of Child	Serial No.	Sex	Date of Birth Day	Month	Year	Age (in months)	Birth cert. Yes/No	Birth order	Months of breast feeding	Weight kg	Height cm	Mid-arm circumference cm	How many meals Yesterday	Normally	Cereal	Cassava, Potatoes	Bananas	Beans	Other vegetables	Meat	Milk
	11	12	13 14	15 16	17 18	19 20	21	22 23	24 25	26 27 28	29 30 31 32	33 34 35	36	37	38	39	40	41	42	43	44
	45	46	47 48	49 50	51 52	53 54	55	56 57	58 59	60 61 62	63 64 65 66	67 68 69	70	71	72	73	74	75	76	77	78
	11	12	13 14	15 16	17 18	19 20	21	22 23	24 25	26 27 28	29 30 31 32	33 34 35	36	37	38	39	40	41	42	43	44
	45	46	47 48	49 50	51 52	53 54	55	56 57	58 59	60 61 62	63 64 65 66	67 68 69	70	71	72	73	74	75	76	77	78
	11	12	13 14	15 16	17 18	19 20	21	22 23	24 25	26 27 28	29 30 31 32	33 34 35	36	37	38	39	40	41	42	43	44

(Frequency of consumption of staple foods [b]: Cereal, Cassava Potatoes, Bananas, Beans, Other vegetables, Meat, Milk)

45	46	47	48	49	50	51	52	53	54	55	56	57	58	59	60	61	62	63	64	65	66	67	68	69	70	71	72	73	74	75	76	77	78
11	12	13	14	15	16	17	18	19	20	21	22	23	24	25	26	27	28	29	30	31	32	33	34	35	36	37	38	39	40	41	42	43	44
45	46	47	48	49	50	51	52	53	54	55	56	57	58	59	60	61	62	63	64	65	66	67	68	69	70	71	72	73	74	75	76	77	78
11	12	13	14	15	16	17	18	19	20	21	22	23	24	25	26	27	28	29	30	31	32	33	34	35	36	37	38	39	40	41	42	43	44
45	46	47	48	49	50	51	52	53	54	55	56	57	58	59	60	61	62	63	64	65	66	67	68	69	70	71	72	73	74	75	76	77	78

a Questionnaire by the Central Bureau of Statistics, Kenya, in the rural survey of 1976-1977 (nutrition module) (15).

b Code frequency: 1: Once a day — 2: Two or more times a day — 3: Two or three times a week — 4: Once a week — 5: Rarely — 6: Never

The criterion of demonstrated need for the data applies in this situation as in any other. Possibly a different audience is reached by data from household surveys, and different institutions are involved, than in the case of systems based on routine administrative data. Hence, different people may need to be convinced of their utility.

Analytical capacity is almost always a crucial constraint. The interpretation of nutritional data may often be unfamiliar to staff regularly engaged in the analysis of household survey data, for example in statistical offices. The potential availability of staff and analytical procedures must be a major consideration in deciding whether to include a nutrition module in a survey. Assistance may be required from local institutions with human resources capable of handling nutritional data.

The choice of the variables to be included in a nutrition module depends partly on the data already available from other parts of the survey. However, it offers a particularly good opportunity to obtain precisely the information required. It may be worth repeating that the following basic outcome indicators are often of particular interest: anthropometric measurements of preschool children; infant and child mortality rates; estimated morbidity; living standards and sanitation (e.g., quality of housing, degree of overcrowding, water supply, sanitary facilities); and access to services. Except for the anthropometric measurements, data on these variables can be obtained by means of a questionnaire to be answered either by the child's mother or by the head of the household, and several of the data may already be included in the basic survey to which the nutrition module is attached. Short-cut questions have been used to estimate mortality and morbidity. For mortality, comparisons between different groups have been made using the questions: "How many children have been born alive in this household, or to this mother? How many are alive now?" Although this approach does not elicit absolute mortality rates – and moreover often reaches only mothers whose children are of preschool age and therefore being measured anthropometrically – it has made it possible to obtain comparative values. The equivalent questions for morbidity are more familiar: "Has the child had fever, or diarrhoea, today/in the last three days/in the last week?" Again comparative data have been obtained with such questions.

The enumerator can obtain data on the physical amenities of the household (e.g., type of housing, water supply, sanitary facilities) by direct observation. Such matters as the roofing material, the number of rooms, etc., as well as the possession of certain consumer durables (e.g., bed, radio) are readily noted.

At the same time as information on selected variables is being collected at the household level, it may be found useful to collect similar information at the village level: Is there a health centre? A school? How far is the village from the nearest road? etc. Although this type of information may be available from other parts of the survey, it is often worth considering its inclusion in the nutrition module for ease of analysis.

References

1. *Development of indicators for monitoring progress towards health for all by the year 2000.* Geneva, World Health Organization, 1981 ("Health for All" Series, No. 4).

2. *Measuring change in nutritional status.* Geneva, World Health Organization, 1983.

3. KELLER, W. ET AL. Anthropometry in nutrition surveillance: a review based on results of the WHO Collaborative Study on Nutritional Anthropometry. *Nutrition abstracts and reviews,* **46**: 591-609 (1976).

4. HABICHT, J.-P. Estandardización de métodos epidemilógicos cuantitativos sobre el terreno. *Boletín de la Oficina Sanitaria Panamericana,* **76**: 375-384 (1974).

5. PUFFER, R. R. & SERRANO, C. V. *Patterns of mortality in childhood.* Washington, DC, Pan American Health Organization, 1973 (Scientific Publication, No. 262).

6. SOMMER, A. & LOEWENSTEIN, M. S. Nutritional status and mortality: a prospective validation of the QUAC stick. *American journal of clinical nutrition,* **28**: 287-292 (1975).

7. CHEN, L. C. ET AL. Anthropometric assessment of energy-protein malnutrition and subsequent risk of mortality among preschool age children. *American journal of clinical nutrition,* **33**: 1836-1845 (1980).

8. KIELMAN, A. A. & McCORD, C. Weight-for-age as an index of risk of death in children. *Lancet,* **1**: 1247-1250 (1978).

9. HABICHT, J.-P. ET AL. Height and weight standards for preschool children: Are there really ethnic differences in growth potential? *Lancet,* **1**: 611-615 (1974).

10. GOMEZ, F. ET AL. Mortality in second and third degree malnutrition. *Journal of tropical pediatrics,* **2**: 77-83 (1956).

11. Classification of infantile malnutrition. *Lancet,* **2**: 302 (1970).

12. WATERLOW, J. C. Note on the assessment and classification of protein-energy malnutrition in children. *Lancet,* **2**: 87-89 (1973).

13. SRI LANKA. MINISTRY OF HEALTH. *Nutrition status survey.* Washington, DC, USAID – Office of Nutrition, 1976.

14. KENYA. CENTRAL BUREAU OF STATISTICS. The Rural Kenyan Nutrition Survey, February-March 1977. *Social perspectives,* **2** (4): 1-32 (1977).

15. KENYA. CENTRAL BUREAU OF STATISTICS. *Child nutrition in rural Kenya.* Nairobi, UNICEF, 1979.

16. UNITED STATES OF AMERICA. NATIONAL CENTER FOR HEALTH STATISTICS. *Vital registration systems in five developing countries: Honduras, Mexico, the Philippines, Thailand and Jamaica.* Hyattsville, MD, NCHS, 1980 (Vital and Health Statistics Series 2, No. 79; DHHS Publication No. (PHS) 81-1353).

17. RUEDA WILLIAMSON, R. ET AL. *Rev. pediatr.,* **10**: 335 (1969).

18. PHILIPPINES. NATIONAL NUTRITION COUNCIL. *Philippine Nutrition Program, Implementing guidelines,* Manila, National Nutrition Council, 1981.

19. ROIG OLLER, J. Estudio de la historia nutricional en Costa Rica mediante el indicador talla/edad. *Boletín informativo del SIN,* **1** (1): 5-7 (1980).

20. VALVERDE, V. Regionalización de los problemas nutricionales y análisis de la talla y la edad de ingreso a primer grado de los niños costaricenses. *Boletín informativo del SIN,* **1** (7): 23-31 (1980).

21. INTERNATIONAL STATISTICAL INSTITUTE. *Manual on sample design.* London, International Statistical Institute, 1975 (World Fertility Survey Basic Documentation, No. 3).

22. EGYPT. MINISTRY OF HEALTH. *National nutrition survey.* Washington, DC, USAID – Office of Nutrition, 1978.

23. UNITED NATIONS. DEPARTMENT OF INTERNATIONAL ECONOMIC AND SOCIAL AFFAIRS. STATISTICAL OFFICE. *The feasibility of welfare-oriented measures to supplement the national accounts and balances: a technical report.* New York, United Nations, 1977 (Studies in Methods, Series F, No. 22; ST/ESA/STAT/SER. F/22).

24. UNITED NATIONS. DEPARTMENT OF INTERNATIONAL ECONOMIC AND SOCIAL AFFAIRS, STATISTICAL OFFICE. *Social indicators: preliminary guidelines and illustrative series.* New York, United Nations, 1978 (Statistical Papers Series M. No. 63; ST/ESA/STAT/SER. M/63).

25. SHEEHAN, G. & HOPKINS, M. *Basic needs performance,* Geneva, International Labour Office, 1979.

26. UNITED NATIONS. DEPARTMENT OF INTERNATIONAL ECONOMIC AND SOCIAL AFFAIRS, STATISTICAL OFFICE. *Compendium of housing statistics, 1975-1977,* 3rd ed. New York, United Nations, 1980.

27. WORLD HEALTH ORGANIZATION. Community water supply and excreta disposal in developing countries. Review of progress. *World health statistics report,* **29**: 544-603 (1976).

28. *The fourth world food survey.* Rome, Food and Agriculture Organization of the United Nations, 1977 (FAO Statistics Series, No. 11; FAO Food and Nutrition Series, No. 10).

29. POLEMAN, T. T. *Quantifying the nutrition situation in developing countries.* Ithaca, NY, Cornell University, 1979 (Cornell Agricultural Economics Staff Paper No. 79-33).

30. POLEMAN, T. T. A reappraisal of the extent of world hunger. *Food policy,* **6**: 236-252 (1981).

31. PEKKANIRENN, M. Methodology in the collection of food consumption data. *World review of nutrition and dietetics,* **12**: 145-171 (1970).

32. LECHTIG, A. ET AL. The one-day recall dietary survey. A review of its usefulness to estimate protein and calorie intake. *Archivos latinamericanos de nutrición,* **26**: 243-271 (1976).

33. VALVERDE, V. ET AL. *The measurement of individuals' food intake in longitudinal nutritional studies in poor rural communities in Guatemala.* Guatemala, Institute of Nutrition of Central America and Panama (INCAP), 1980.

34. MORRIS, M. D. *Measuring the condition of the world's poor. The Physical Quality of Life Index.* London & New York, Pergamon Press, 1979 (Pergamon Policy Studies No. 42).

35. WHO Technical Report Series, No. 593, 1976 *(Methodology of nutritional surveillance. Report of a Joint FAO/UNICEF/WHO Expert Committee).*

36. *Health programme evaluation. Guiding principles for its application in the managerial process for national health development.* Geneva, World Health Organization, 1981 (''Health for All'' Series, No. 6).

37. CASLEY, D. J. & LURY, D. A. *A handbook on monitoring and evaluation of agricultural and rural development projects.* Washington, DC, World Bank, 1981.

38. SNEDECOR, G. W. & COCHRAN, W. G. *Statistical methods,* 7th ed., Ames, Iowa State University Press, 1980.

39. TROWBRIDGE, F. ET AL. Evaluation of nutrition surveillance indicators. *Bulletin of the Pan American Health Organization,* **14**: 238-243 (1980).

40. INDIA. VITAL STATISTICS DIVISION, OFFICE OF THE REGISTRAR GENERAL. *Civil registration system in India – a perspective.* New Delhi, Ministry of Home Affairs, 1972 (Census Centenary Monograph No. 4).

41. WHO Technical Report Series, No. 559, 1974 *(New approaches in health statistics. Report of the Second International Conference of National Committees on Vital and Health Statistics).*

42. PHILIPPINES. NATIONAL NUTRITION COUNCIL. *The Philippine Nutrition Program 1978-1982.* Manila, National Nutrition Council, 1977.

43. PHILIPPINES. *First nationwide nutrition survey – Philippines, 1978* Manila, Food and Nutrition Research Institute, 1980 (FNRI Publication No. GP-11).

44. UNITED NATIONS. DEPARTMENT OF INTERNATIONAL ECONOMIC AND SOCIAL AFFAIRS. STATISTICAL OFFICE. *Studies in the integration of social statistics: technical report.* New York, United Nations, 1979 (Studies in Methods, Series F, No. 24 ST/ESA/STAT/SER. F/24).

45. UNITED NATIONS. DEPARTMENT OF INTERNATIONAL ECONOMIC AND SOCIAL AFFAIRS. STATISTICAL OFFICE. *The National Household Survey Capability Programme. Prospectus.* New York, United Nations, 1980 (DP/UN/INT-79-020/1).

46. CASLEY, D. & LURY, D. *Data collection in developing countries.* London & New York, Oxford University Press, 1981.

47. VALVERDE, V. ET AL. Organization of an information system for food and nutrition programmes in Costa Rica. *Food and nutrition,* **7**: 32-40 (1981).

48. CHILE. CONPAN. *Chile: Estadísticas básicas en alimentación y nutrición, 1969-1978.* Santiago, Ministerio de Salud, 1980.

49. HAKIM, P. & SOLIMANO, G. *Development, reform, and malnutrition in Chile.* Cambridge, MA, MIT Press, 1978.

50. TAUCHER, E. La mortalidad infantil en Chile. *Notas de población,* **7**: 35-72 (1979).

51. UNICEF. *Social statistics programme. Child mortality in Kenya. Series of 4 maps based on 1979 census estimates.* Nairobi, UNICEF.

52. UNITED NATIONS. DEPARTMENT OF INTERNATIONAL ECONOMIC AND SOCIAL AFFAIRS, STATISTICAL OFFICE. *1978 report on the world social situation.* New York, United Nations, 1979 (Publication E/CN.5/557.ST/ESA/87).

53. KENYA. CENTRAL BUREAU OF STATISTICS. *Integrated rural survey 1974-75. Basic report.* Nairobi, Central Bureau of Statistics, 1977.

54. COSTA RICA. SISTEMA DE INFORMACIÓN EN NUTRICIÓN. *Encuesta nacional de nutrición, 1978. Aspectos socioeconómicos de la nutrición.* San José, Oficina de Información, Casa Presidencial, 1980.

55. PERISSE, J. & KAMOUN, A. The price of satiety: a study of household consumption budgets in Tunisia. *Food and nutrition,* **7**: 3-10 (1981).

56. UNITED STATES OF AMERICA. NATIONAL CENTER FOR HEALTH STATISTICS. NCHS growth charts, 1976. *Monthly vital statistics report,* **25** (3), Suppl. (HRA) 76-1120 (1976).

57. MASON, J. B. *Case-study for FAO on introducing nutrition considerations into development project planning - Haiti.* Rome, Food and Agriculture Organization of the United Nations, 1983.

58. VALVERDE, V. ET AL. Relación entre la prevalencia de retardo en talla en escolares e indicadores socioeconómics a nivel de canton en Costa Rica. *Boletín informativo del SIN,* **2** (10): 4-10 (1980).

59. *World development report, 1979.* Washington, DC, World Bank, 1979, pp. 117-188 (Annex: World development indicators).

60. CHAVERRI, G. & VALVERDE, V. Evolución de los salarios mínimos en Costa Rica en relación a precios de alimentos durante la decada de 1970. *Boletín informativo del SIN,* **1** (9) 11-20 (1980).

CHAPTER 5

Nutritional surveillance for programme management and evaluation

Summary

Nutritional surveillance methods can be adapted for regular monitoring and evaluation of the adequacy of programmes as part of their routine management. This chapter gives some principles additional to those in Chapter 3 relevant to the use of nutritional surveillance methods for ongoing evaluation. Such evaluation covers both monitoring the process of implementation, particularly targeting, and monitoring the outcome using nutritional indicators. The gross outcome is distinct from the net outcome or impact; impact makes allowance for changes in outcome that would have occurred without the programme. Gross outcome does not make this allowance, but can be used for assessing the adequacy of programmes – hence the term ''adequacy evaluation'' – and for this purpose nutritional surveillance methods are suitable. Adequacy evaluation poses two questions:

1. Is the programme being delivered as planned to the intended target group?
2. Is the gross outcome acceptable?

It emphasizes both process (i.e., programme delivery) and outcome (i.e., change in nutritional status).

Management decisions, based on adequacy evaluation, concern ensuring delivery of the programme to the intended target group; and reassessing delivery and the underlying assumptions if the gross outcome is found to be inadequate. These decisions all relate to the objectives of the programme, and hence to the criteria for adequacy set in the programme planning. The quantities in terms of which the objectives are set become the indicators for adequacy evaluation. In setting these objectives, two aspects require particular emphasis: specification of target groups and deciding expected changes in outcome variables. Specifying target groups using baseline data involves deciding on planned coverage and focusing on those most in need of the programme. Monitoring then includes measuring actual coverage and the extent to which focusing has succeeded, as well as assessing delivery and leakage. Outcome objectives may be set as a range of values, deviation below the lower limit of which indicates inadequacy. The basis for deciding adequacy levels for outcome is discussed. Common outcome indicators are pointed out, anthropometric variables being the most widely used.

Organization for ongoing adequacy evaluation requires clear assignment of responsibilities for decisions, for managing the evaluation, and for data collection, processing and analysis. Various possibilities for organization of data collection are discussed: from programme contacts, administrative sources, community weighing programmes, and special purpose surveys – either separately or as part of broader evaluation surveys.

Examples are given of two nutrition programme evaluations that approximate to these concepts. Finally, experience of the monitoring and evaluation of development programmes is extensive and relevant, and is briefly reviewed. It suggests that nutritional variables – which are becoming accepted as a measure of socioeconomic development – and methods of nutritional surveillance may be useful in this area.

Introduction

Policies for improving nutrition lead to specific programmes – both those with nutrition as their main objective (e.g., public health, feeding programmes), and those whose objectives include better satisfaction of the basic needs of the poor (e.g., rural development programmes). Nutrition information is required for the design and management of these programmes. The information described in the previous chapters (3 and 4) indicates in general terms where, and for whom, programmes are needed, and their likely effects on nutritional outcome. But when it comes to designing a particular programme, and monitoring its effects for management purposes, more detailed and programme-specific data are needed, often in a different organizational setting, leading to different decisions.

The main focus here is on regular monitoring and evaluation of the adequacy of programmes as part of their routine management. Nutritional surveillance methods are suited to this function. The data produced may also contribute to evaluation of the impact of a programme, and hence to more far-reaching policy decisions.

The methods of nutritional surveillance given in Chapters 3 and 4 are applicable to ongoing programme evaluation, with certain essential adaptations. This chapter gives the *additional* principles involved and does not repeat those aspects already discussed. As before, the methods apply both to interventions conventionally planned with nutritional improvement as the primary objective – usually nutrition and primary health care programmes – and to development programmes with the more general objective of improving the satisfaction of basic needs. Much of what is given below relates to giving operational effect to the concepts laid out in *Health programme evaluation (1)*.

Purposes of Evaluation

The question of interest in programme management is: "Is the programme going as intended?" Answers to this question are needed to enable programme management to decide whether to:
- tighten up on management of present procedures;
- change procedures to improve activities;
- change or institute new activities to improve results.

This question is more limited than those usually asked by those responsible for overall administration of a number of programmes and for funding a programme. They are typically concerned also with whether to:
- continue the programme;
- maintain the same activities with fewer resources;
- seek the same results with fewer resources;
- provide more resources for new or different activities in the same area;
- expand the programme to new, dissimilar areas.

Table 5.1. Steps in programme evaluation

Step	Information required
A. What is evaluation for? (desk)	1. For whom intended (who are the principals)? For what decisions? 2. What objectives of the programme are to be evaluated? = Required cooperative venture between evaluators and principals → consensus regarding explicit objectives and resolution of contradictions. 3. What are supposed to be the programme procedures and activities? = Original plan + changes → consensus regarding explicit procedures and activities. 4. Plan the evaluation.
B. Is the programme design likely to meet programme objectives? (desk)	1. Objectives: What impacts are sought? In whom? May vary with impact sought → define "adequate outcome". 2. Activities: Will designed activities attain objectives in those who receive them? 3. Targeting: Will planned targeting attain objectives in population? 4. Procedures: Will designed procedures result in activities and targeting planned? 5. Estimate effects and cost/effect: Are they adequate and reasonable? 6. Reiterate steps 1–5 until consensus reached. 7. If answer to any question 2–5 is "No", do not proceed further.
C. Is the programme implementation likely to meet the objectives? (field)	1. Is implementation of delivery as designed? 2. Is implementation of targeting as designed? 3. Do deviations in procedures affect activities? 4. Are deviations in activities likely to prevent attainment of outcome objectives? 5. If answer to 4 is "Yes", do not proceed to evaluation of those outcomes. 6. What are constraints on implementation? Can they be remedied? 7. If answer to 6 is "No", this answers all other questions.

D. What is gross outcome? (field: quantitative measurements)	1. Outcome in whom? Needy
	                      Targeted
	                      Recipients
	                      Total population
	2. Adequacy of attained outcome (needs standard)
	3. If inadequate, would nutritional situation be likely to be significantly worse without the programme? (negative confounding)
	4. Upper limit of cost-effectiveness – if too high and no negative confounding likely, stop programme.

E. What is net impact?	1. Gross difference in double-blind randomized trial = net impact.
	2. Gross difference outcome + attempted discarding of confounding = approximate net impact.
	3. Cost-effectiveness = true net impact per unit cost
	  • Differentiate between effect on variable in individual and adequacy of effect in individual
	  • In whom?
	    — cost-effectiveness improves with increase in individual's need (responsiveness) and prevalence of need among those covered, but decreases with success.

F. Data presentation and distribution	1. To whom? Already prepared – principals (manager and funder) should have been involved in draft of report.
	2. What type of presentation? Frequent iterative presentations improve the usefulness of the report by better addressing the needs of the recipient, both as to what is addressed and how it is done.
	3. Feedback to other than principals?
	    ● Do it in collaboration with principals (respect ethics of confidentiality and censorship)
	    ● Busy people need short summaries of decision options + results + recommendations. Careful people need everything relevant – fill these two needs separately.

Finally, research is usually concerned with cause-effect relations between programme activities and outcome, in order to design new programmes or modify the design of existing ones.

The term "evaluation" has been used when addressing all the above questions. However, the answers required for management are less demanding in their data and analytical needs, and the methods of nutritional surveillance described in Chapters 3 and 4 can be adapted for these purposes. These methods are most effective when used regularly for ongoing evaluation. Programme evaluations dealing with all the above questions have been described elsewhere, by ourselves (2, 3) and others. The principal steps are set out in Table 5.1. – adapted from ref. 3. The questions that are the concerns of programme management – which are a subset of all evaluation concerns – are the subject of this chapter. They are summarized in steps C and D of Table 5.1. Steps A and B are obvious prerequisites, not treated in detail here. Step E – evaluating net impact – is usually beyond the scope of nutritional surveillance methods and of programme management.

Experience shows that those involved in a programme have different expectations about the purpose and results of evaluation. It is important that the decisions for which the evaluation is being done be clearly understood and agreed upon. The design of the evaluation must then be tailored to this purpose, and the presentation of the results must be matched to it. For instance, results presented as if the purpose is to decide the continuation or termination of a programme are inappropriate, if the purpose of the evaluation is to improve the programme. Here we are primarily concerned with methods that can improve the programme, hence usually with evaluation built into the management of the programme. This is in line with the priorities for health programme evaluation set out by WHO (1, pp. 11,15). Before proceeding, we need to define certain important terms used throughout.

It is necessary to distinguish in the first instance between project implementation itself and the effects of this implementation. This broadly divides the subject into *process* and *outcome*. A further common distinction (used for example by the World Bank (*4*)) is that into inputs and outputs (i.e., process); and effects and impact (i.e., outcome). Overlapping concepts in the evaluation literature (*5*) are: formative evaluation, which results in changes in a programme to improve it (in practice this is usually called process evaluation); and summative evaluation to see what is the overall result (outcome evaluation).

Process

Monitoring of programme procedures and activities, known as process monitoring and/or evaluation, is far more common than monitoring of outcome, and is readily understood. The information under this heading includes:

– procedures to attain activities;
– activities for delivering supplies and services in adequate quality and quantity and for targeting beneficiaries;
– costs, calculated as cost per activity, cost per recipient, cost per recipient who can benefit, etc.

Outcome

There is a crucial difference between "gross outcome" and "net outcome" or "net effects". The latter two terms are synonymous with "impact". Gross outcome refers to changes detected in the population monitored (e.g., changes in nutritional status), but does not relate these to programme activities, since it does not allow for changes in the outcome that might have occurred anyway. This concept is essential to the methods that follow, and is worth a brief digression.

Formally it can be represented as follows:

			1. Endogenous change
Net outcome			2. Secular drift
or			3. Interfering events
Net effects	=	Gross outcome *minus*	4. Maturational trends
or			5. Self-selection
Impact			6. Regression artefacts
			7. Other effects

(See ref. *6*, p. 115; a definition of confounding factors (endogenous change, etc.) is given on pp. 111–114 of this reference; see also ref. *7* for a similar classification.)

The research methods required to take into account confounding factors (e.g., self-selection, interfering events) so as to be able to draw inferences regarding the probability of a net outcome or impact are virtually never feasible in operational programmes. These methods actively randomize confounding factors across the recipients of the programme activities (treatment group) and a control group through random assignment of persons or groups to treatment or control activities (9). This process includes preventing biases in response and measurement by "blinding", i.e., withholding knowledge about who does and does not receive the treatment from both the recipient and the measurers of outcome. This double-blind randomized design is the *only* one that delivers a probability statement that the observed outcome is an impact. Other methods deliver probability statements and demonstrate associations (programme activities are associated with an outcome) but permit no inferences as to causality because the association between activity and outcome could still be due to a confounding factor (e.g., self-selection). Statistical techniques, coupled to the measurements of confounding factors and to quasi-experimental designs (8), can raise the plausibility that one has taken care of confounding before inferring that an association is causal. Such a plausibility statement is unquantifiable (in contrast to a probability statement; e.g., $P < 0.05$), the degree of plausibility depending on how far knowledgeable people feel that confounding has been accounted for.

Most of the information now becoming available from evaluations of nutrition and health programmes is from studies using the above research techniques, i.e., they are impact assessments of pilot-scale projects (see ref. *9-13*). The results summarized in these reviews are important as one basis for deciding what changes in outcome might be considered adequate, but the techniques used are not generally applicable to surveillance.

Gross outcome is much easier to estimate than net outcome using methods applicable to surveillance. Estimation of net outcome requires a full-scale evaluation using the research techniques referred to above. As stated, this is not feasible, at least not regularly, in most operational programmes. On the other hand, monitoring of gross outcome using nutritional surveillance methods may be both feasible and useful, and can contribute to "adequacy evaluation", the definition of which is discussed below. An example of monitoring gross outcome could be as follows. A supplementary feeding programme involves delivery of food to mothers of preschool children attending a clinic. The children are periodically weighed, which allows estimation of whether their nutritional status is improving. This change in nutritional status is the gross outcome in this target group and may represent important information for those running the programme, even though it does not allow estimation of the extent to which the programme itself has caused any changes, since the change in outcome that would have taken place without the programme is not estimated.

Adequacy evaluation

Evaluation of the adequacy of a programme covers both process and outcome. It is essentially concerned with two questions:

(*a*) Is the programme being delivered as planned to the intended target group?

(*b*) Is the (gross) outcome acceptable?

Adequacy evaluation uses gross outcome, in contrast to impact assessment, which uses net outcome.

The second question could be elaborated as: Is the trend in outcome indicators adequate for the programme target groups *or* in the population as a whole?

A diagram summarizing the steps involved in adequacy evaluation is given in Fig. 5.1. (It should be noted that the definition of adequacy used here extends that used in *Health programme evaluation* (*1*, p. 29) to satisfactory programme performance.)

There are two requirements for adequacy evaluation. First, a clear and quantified definition of the target groups is needed. Second, a definition of adequacy is needed; this involves both defining the units in which procedures, activities (i.e., process) and outcomes are to be measured, and setting levels of these units, any deviation from which will be considered evidence of inadequacy

Fig. 5.1. Adequacy-evaluation framework

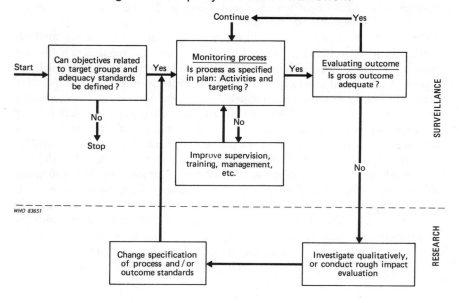

and will lead to further action. Both these requirements are met in the planning stage.

Adequacy evaluation can derive costs relative to procedures and activities, and costs relative to gross outcome, either for the programme target group or in the population as a whole. It will not be possible to derive a true estimate of cost-effectiveness, meaning cost per unit of net outcome *due to the project*.

Adequacy evaluation should take off from the point at which the necessary experiments and pilot trials have been made in order to determine that, on the experimental scale, a particular intervention is effective, i.e., at the point at which it is intended to expand to wider operations. At all events, the evaluation methods cannot be a substitute for such research, even if the research was not in fact done and it is decided to implement a programme anyway. A desirable sequence of events in research, planning and evaluation (for nutrition and public health programmes) is set out by Habicht (*14*). This may not always be followed (maybe for good reason), particularly with regard to the nutritional effects of development programmes; in this case less rigorous sequences may still give useful answers. However, if the assumption can be made that a particular programme *should* have a positive effect on the nutrition of the participants – an assumption that does, in fact, apply in many cases – an evaluation for adequacy of the programme will be easier. This is tantamount to saying that adequacy evaluation applies when improvement in nutrition is an objective of the programme, and when the planning has explicitly taken this into account. Further, its usefulness depends on linking the information to management decisions.

Below, we first discuss the management decisions that can result from adequacy evaluation. These depend in turn on the programmes objectives, and the means of setting these objectives are discussed in the subsequent section.

Management Decisions

The decisions available from adequacy evaluation are primarily relevant to management of the programme itself.

Decisions from process data – one product of adequacy evaluation – relate to two main questions:

1. Is the actual delivery to recipients of programme services, resources, etc. of acceptable quantity and quality in relation to the work-plan? (Question C-1, Table 5.1). This aspect of evaluation may serve in the first instance to highlight problems and hence stimulate action.

2. Are the recipients of services, resources, etc. the intended target group? (Question C-2, Table 5.1). Failure in this respect will usually mean that the possibility of the outcome reaching adequacy is diminished, either because the programme benefits the less needy, so that resources are withdrawn from those in need, or because the planned chain of events leading to the intended outcome will be interrupted. Outcome may be specified either for direct participants or

for a larger population group. In either case, however, deviation in delivery from the specified target groups is likely to affect outcome.

Two decisions could be based on the information that either of the above aspects of programme delivery is unsatisfactory in reaching the intended target group. The first would be simply to improve the management and organization of the programme. However, there is a second possibility that the planned means of identifying target populations and delivering services to them did not turn out to be practical (Question C-6, Table 5.1). This should lead to a reassessment of the project design, including the implications for likely outcome and its cost-effectiveness. In many cases, failures in one or other of these areas is likely to account for inadequacy of outcome.

The hoped-for decision based on outcome data (Questions D1-6, Table 5.1) is that they indicate adequacy and that the programme should continue as it is. Because decisions may otherwise be difficult to take, it is important to pre-establish levels of adequacy, and to use these to trigger action methods for setting adequacy levels are given in the next section). The first step following the decision that outcome indicators are *inadequate* will be to investigate the reasons. The data available from the monitoring may not always help in establishing these reasons, and *ad hoc* investigations may be required. There are only a limited number of possible reasons for inadequate outcome, as follows:

1. The process of programme delivery may be inadequate, although not detected as being so from process evaluation. The first step is therefore likely to be re-examination of programme delivery.

2. Some intermediate step between delivery and outcome is not operating as expected. An obvious example might be a take-home feeding programme with the goal of increasing the weight of preschool children. The project may monitor the delivery of food to the family and the weight of the child whose growth is to be improved. Here, the input of services monitored is one step away from the intended outcome. The food does reach the household, but it may not reach the child in the form or quantity intended, if the parents use it to feed others in the family or sell it to purchase other goods. In this case, measurement of implementation could be inadequate, and the problem would only show up in measuring outcome. This type of effect accounts for many of the results given by Beaton & Ghassemi (10). Determining that such an explanation was valid could require additional data collection.

3. The assumptions underlying the project design are wrong. An example might be from a programme designed to provide a protein supplement to children to prevent protein-energy malnutrition, when the actual dietary deficiency was primarily of total energy. Such findings might not show up in pilot trials – especially if the situation of the programme participants alters during the programme. A conclusion based on the underlying assumptions should evidently lead to a decision to redesign the project. But it must be clear that the evaluation methods discussed here are not appropriate for testing these assumptions scientifically. That requires ascertainment of net impact.

4. Factors external to the programme are causing a deterioration in outcome indicators in the population as a whole. An epidemic, price inflation, drought, or other factors could be involved. If these were shown to exist – probably by using data from outside the programme area – then the adequacy criteria themselves would need to be re-evaluated. For example, the programme might be justified as mitigating or preventing deterioration. The possible effects of external factors may in some cases be assessed by the programme management. This requires an assessment of whether the nutrition of those not participating in the programme has deteriorated, unless it is postulated that the detrimental factors only affect programme participants. Evidence is likely to be available to support such conclusions from sources other than the programme itself. Closer examination may again require an impact assessment, taking confounding factors quantitatively into account.

In the examples 2–4 the design now needs to be looked at. This may go beyond the capabilities of programme management, and it may be decided to bring in, for instance, those concerned with the programme planning itself to reassess the programme – along the lines of step B, Table 5.1. This reassessment goes beyond considerations of surveillance and is not further discussed.

The flow of management decisions described above is summarized in Fig. 5.1, which also introduces the concepts of setting objectives and adequacy standards. These are discussed in the next section.

Setting Objectives and Choosing Indicators

All decisions relate to the objectives of the programme. Programme evaluation needs to be made against stated programme objectives or criteria (see Table 5.1, Step B–1). These objectives again involve both process and outcome. The objectives of the programme must be explicit and should be understood and agreed upon by those who must use the results of the evaluation to make management decisions. Once the objectives of the programme and the purpose of the evaluation are defined, one should translate the objectives into some expected outcome, expressed in quantitative terms, such as a change in the prevalence of malnutrition. This is equivalent to setting criteria, as defined in ref. *1*, p. 6. The quantities in which the objectives are set become the indicators for adequacy evaluation. An *a priori* calculation of expected costs relative to expected effects should be made as part of setting objectives. This then leads to defining the goods and services that will be provided to the target group in order to bring about the expected improvements.

Two particular objectives for which calculations should be made require some additional theory:

– specification of target groups (included in process objectives);

– expected changes in outcome variables (e.g., nutritional status) of target groups (outcome objectives).

Process

Definition of activities

The definition of activities to be monitored in process evaluation depends on the specifics of the programme. Typical process objectives, and hence measurements in many nutrition/health programmes, concern the following:

1. Timing of delivery supplies and equipment.
2. Participation of target groups:
   (*a*) by attendance;
   (*b*) by receipt of food, immunization, health care, health and nutrition education, etc.
3. Staff performance:
   (*a*) contacts with recipients per worker;
   (*b*) contact hours per worker.

Management records (e.g., inventory control, supervisory data, finances) should provide data on implementation. The definition of indicators of delivery depends on the specifics of the programme, but is straightforward in principle.

Definition of target groups

Target groups are defined in programme planning in the first instance in order to work out details of the programme itself. That is, it is necessary to calculate how many people will be involved, who they are, where they live, etc., in order to cost programme components and estimate likely effects. In programmes with primarily economic objectives, such information is needed anyway for cost–benefit analysis for assessment of the economic viability of the programme. In such cases – e.g., rural development programmes – target groups will generally be defined by geographical area and by factors such as their production system (crops grown, land-holding, etc.). For more narrowly focused programmes – e.g., nutrition/health – the definition is in terms of area and sometimes need – e.g., number of malnourished children in certain villages.

Baseline information may be required for the selection of target groups. First it is necessary to estimate the number of households or individuals it is intended to reach in the programme. Second, an assessment of relative need may be used in the planning in order to direct programme activities to those with the greatest need, so as to increase the efficiency of the programme. The actual figures used to quantify the population of target groups are usually taken from census data, surveys, local administrative records, etc.

Using this as a basis for adequacy evaluation will require that the definitions used be monitored in practice. For example, if malnourished children in certain villages were targeted, it would be necessary not only to include assessment of the nutritional status of entrants into the programme, but to ensure that these results were reported for monitoring purposes. A second example might be that of a rural development project in which small farmers, defined by land-holding, were targeted; for monitoring purposes data on land-holding areas would then be needed. In the latter case modification of the definition of target group might be needed for monitoring, if land-holding areas were not readily available.

In setting objectives for target groups, and subsequently monitoring programme delivery to these, a number of different groups need to be distinguished. These will vary conceptually depending on the type of programme. The main groups are:

(a) the total population in the programme area;

(b) the population targeted by the programme;

(c) the population in need of better nutrition – called "needy" here (i.e., restricting the term to nutritional need for these purposes);

(d) the population receiving benefits from the programme – called "recipients" here.

In some cases, additional subgroups might need to be considered:

(e) the needy who *could* benefit from the programme; examples of the needy who could not benefit might be malnourished children in a supplementary feeding programme whose nutritional problem is due to malabsorption and not to inadequate food intake; or farming families in an agricultural inputs programme whose main constraint is land availability or tenure (clearly the closer the intervention is matched to the specific cause, the closer the needy population equals the needy who can benefit);

(f) the non-needy who could benefit: whereas well-nourished children might not respond to supplementary feeding, better-off farmers would still benefit from, say, a rural development programme.

It is essential to distinguish between groups (a)–(d), both in planning and in monitoring. The distinction is important conceptually in planning: an overall objective could be stated as reduction of, say, malnutrition in the population as a whole, and targeting used to focus resources on groups with a high prevalence of malnutrition, so as to improve efficiency; on the other hand, the objective could be stated as specifically to improve nutrition only in the target group. It is suggested that the outcome for the planned target group is usually the objective of interest; this objective is sensitive to any deviation in programme delivery to the target group.

Targeting, both in planning and monitoring programme implementation, is concerned with several criteria which must be balanced. In the first place, any programme is likely to be aimed at providing good coverage of those in need, as far as resources permit. In the second place, the aim of targeting is usually to focus resources on those most in need: at a minimum, it is often intended to direct the programme to areas and people worse off than the average for the population as a whole. These concepts can be quantified when certain baseline

Table 5.2. Indicators of targeting and programme delivery

A. Indicators of focusing and coverage, [a] to be calculated during programme planning

		Needy? (e.g., malnourished)		
		YES	NO	
Targeted?	YES	a_1	b_1	Requires baseline data
	NO	c_1	d_1	

Planned focusing:
  Proportion of total targeted that are needy $= \dfrac{a_1}{a_1 + b_1}$

Planned coverage:
  Proportion of total needy that are targeted $= \dfrac{a_1}{a_1 + c_1}$

B. Indicators of leakage and delivery of the programme to be calculated during programme evaluation

		Targeted?		
		YES	NO	
Recipients?	YES	a_2	b_2	– Data from programme contacts
	NO	c_2	d_2	– Requires survey data

Leakage
  Proportion of total recipients targeted $= \dfrac{a_2}{a_2 + b_2}$

  Proportion of total recipients not targeted $= \dfrac{b_2}{a_2 + c_2}$

Delivery
  Proportion of total targeted not recipients $= \dfrac{c_2}{a_2 + c_2}$

  Proportion of total targeted who are recipients $= \dfrac{a_2}{a_2 + c_2}$

[a] In epidemiological terms, focusing is equivalent to positive predictive value; coverage is equivalent to sensitivity.

C. Indicators of focusing and coverage to be calculated during programme evaluation

		Needy?		
		YES	NO	
Recipients?	YES	a_3	b_3	– Data from programme contacts
	NO	c_3	d_3	– Requires survey data

Actual focusing:
Proportion of total recipients who are needy $= \dfrac{a_3}{a_3 + b_3}$

Actual coverage:
Proportion of total needy who are recipients $= \dfrac{a_3}{a_3 + c_3}$

(With delivery exactly as targeted, recipients = targeted, and this table is exactly as Table A)

data are available. They form the basis both for planning, to define "planned coverage" and "planned focusing", and for monitoring, to assess "actual coverage" and "actual focusing", thus measuring deviation from planned targeting. In the third place, during programme implementation there is concern to ensure programme delivery to all, or as many as possible, of those targeted; or conversely, to ensure that the minimum of those targeted are missed. Fourthly, leakage to those not targeted is usually to be avoided.

These concepts are conveniently expressed as three 2×2 tables as shown in Table 5.2 A–C. This representation can provide a basis for monitoring the effectiveness of targeting and delivery.

Table 5.2 A should be drawn up during the programme planning, and requires baseline data. The indicators are:

(a) Proportion of total needy that are targeted, reflecting planned coverage of the programme.

(b) Proportion of total targeted that are needy (needy in this case could be, for example, households with children of less than 80% weight-for-age), indicating the degree of planned focusing of the programme towards nutrition. If the prevalence of malnutrition in the population is 30%, the aim will be to have a target group in which the prevalence is greater than 30%, if targeting is designed to direct resources preferentially to the malnourished. (In programmes with a screening procedure, the aim may be to admit to the programme *all* those who are needy, in which case the planned focusing is 100%, i.e., $c_1 = 0$ in Table 5.2A.)

Table 5.3. Example of calculations from Table 5.2.

Consider a district-level programme that could be targeted to two sub-areas in the district.
Suppose Area A has 60% malnutrition (e.g. households with children of less than 80% weight-for-age) and 5 000 households; and area B has 30% malnutrition, 4 000 households. If A is made the target area, 3 000 "needy" households are targeted, plus 2 000 "non-needy"; 1 200 "needy" households are not targeted in area B. Table 5.2A becomes:

		Needy?		TOTALS
		YES	NO	
Targeted?	YES	3 000	2 000	5 000 = Area A
	NO	1 200	2 800	4 000 = Area B
		4 200	4 800	

Planned focusing:
   proportion of total targeted who are needy $= \dfrac{3\,000}{5\,000} = 60\%$

Planned coverage:
   proportion of total needy that are targeted $= \dfrac{3\,000}{4\,200} = 71\%$

If targeting were 100% effective − i.e., only area A actually received the programme, Table 5.2B becomes:

		Targeted?		
		YES	NO	
Recipients?	YES	5 000	0	5 000
	NO	0	4 000	4 000
		5 000	4 000	

and Table 5.2C becomes equivalent to A, i.e.:

		Needy?		
		YES	NO	
Recipients?	YES	3 000	2 000	5 000
	NO	1 200	2 800	4 000
		4 200	4 800	

If, on the other hand, 60% of the population in area A was reached, and 40% in area B, Table 5.2B would become:

		Targeted?		
		YES	NO	
Recipients?	YES	3 000	1 600	4 600
	NO	2 000	2 400	4 400
		5 000	4 000	

Leakage: proportion of total recipients not targeted $= \dfrac{1\ 600}{4\ 600} = 35\%$

Delivery: proportion of total targeted that are recipients $= \dfrac{3\ 000}{5\ 000} = 60\%$

and Table 5.2C becomes:

		Needy?		
		YES	NO	
Recipients?	YES	2 280	2 320	4 600
	NO	1 920	2 480	4 400
		4 200	4 800	

Actual focusing: proportion of total recipients who are needy $= \dfrac{2\ 280}{4\ 600} = 50\%$

(compare with population prevalence of needy $= 47\%$)

Actual coverage: proportion of total needy who are recipients $= \dfrac{2\ 280}{4\ 200} = 54\%$

Table 5.2B provides indicators for evaluation designed to define accuracy of delivery to the target group and leakage to the non-targeted population. Indicators of efficiency of programme delivery could be:

(a) Proportion of total recipients targeted or, conversely, proportion of total recipients not targeted (leakage). These ratios can be derived from data obtained from programme recipients only and do not require baseline data, in contrast to (b).

(b) Proportion of total targeted population who are recipients (delivery) or, conversely, proportion of total targeted population who are not recipients. These ratios require the value c_2 in Table 5.2B, i.e., the number of those targeted who are *not* receiving the programme. This value can be obtained by difference if the total number of persons targeted is known from baseline data (i.e., $a_2 + c_2$, which equals $a_1 + b_1$).

Data presented as in Table 5.2C allow monitoring of the extent to which the needy are actually covered, this table thus performing an analogous function to Table 5.2A in the planning stage. It provides indicators such as:

(a) Proportion of total recipients who are needy (actual focusing). This ratio can be calculated from data obtained on programme recipients only.

(b) Proportion of total needy who are recipients (actual coverage). This ratio requires baseline data on total numbers of needy.

Since in Table 5.2, $a_1 + b_1 = a_2 + c_2$ and $a_1 + c_1 = a_3 + c_3$, baseline data together with data derived from programme delivery to recipients will allow calculation of all the figures in Tables 5.2A, B and C. This has important implications concerning the need for survey data in project monitoring, as discussed in the next section. A worked example is given in Table 5.3.

Outcome

Whereas process objectives and indicators are dictated by the programme design itself, outcome objectives and indicators require both a knowledge of the probable effects of a programme and a careful initial statement as to *why* the programme is being carried out in the first place. Moreover, outcome indicators may not always be directly related to the objective – they may be proxies: for example, a maternal and child health programme could well have improved maternal nutrition and decreased infant mortality as objectives, but for practical reasons evaluation of progress might rely primarily on estimates of birth weight. In a recent review (2) of indicators actually used in relation to objectives, we found that anthropometric indicators were the most widely used among many others suggested. They will be used here for illustrations of nutrition and health projects. Food consumption is also considered with respect to development programmes. Finally, a brief summary of common nutritional outcome indicators is given.

Expected outcomes from nutrition and health programmes

As far as we know, there is no agreed method at present for deciding the extent to which nutrition is expected to improve, on a community basis, as a result of any nutrition or health intervention. There is, however, accumulating evidence that detectable changes do occur. A considerable number of carefully observed pilot projects have been carried out over the last several years (see ref. *13*, pp. 45-47). However, it is probably too early to postulate changes quantitatively in nutrition resulting from defined inputs – at least, this has not been done. Almost all the results used in attempting to evaluate nutrition and health interventions are from studies with substantial research inputs, and problems of scaling-up are well-known (*15*); hence, the results may not, perhaps, be easily generalized to routine programme delivery. Results have been put together by Gwatkin et al. (*11*) and Drake et al. (*12*), generally from combined health care/nutrition programmes. Habicht & Butz (*9*) summarized results from supplementary feeding projects. Beaton & Ghassemi have summarized the way in which 44 food distribution programmes have been evaluated, and concluded that "...most studies have demonstrated some degree of benefit measured in anthropometric terms... The benefit is not always large for the group as a whole... a good number of programes appear to have had little or no impact on the total intervention population..." (*10*, p. 882). Results such as these could be extremely useful in allowing some estimate to be made of the approximate degree of change to be expected if a nutrition/health programme is delivered as planned.

Here we give a brief summary of the sort of changes in nutrition it might be reasonable to expect from different programmes. This is intended only for very rough guidance, and is put forward partly because the absence (as far as we know) of any such guidance in the literature perhaps shows excessive caution in view of recent substantial investment in evaluations.

Recent reviews of evaluations of the gross outcomes of a number *of nutrition/ public health* projects seem to show some consistency in the results. The projects apparently achieved a reduction of around 5-15 cases per 100 in the prevalence of malnutrition, or an improvement of about 2-6% in mean weight-for-age. The time periods vary, as does whether the effects are measured on the target population as a whole or only on those individuals who participated fully in the projects. Nor is it considered in principle whether (*a*) we should expect a continued improvement in outcome indicators of nutritional status over the duration of the programme, or whether there comes a time where no further improvement could be expected; or (*b*) the improvement once attained can be expected to continue if the programme ceases. None the less, a bracketing of expected effects is feasible, and figures of a reduction in prevalence of 5-15 cases per 100 over one or two years would not be an unreasonable mid-point for interventions when the initial prevalences are of the order 30%.

Expected outcomes from income-generating programmes

The effects of income on nutritional status operate substantially through food consumption. However, the relation between changes in food consumption and changes in nutritional status in quantitative terms is also virtually unknown, though some relation can be assumed. It is therefore pertinent to consider rates of change in income, for which data may be available, as offering a rough guide to changes in food consumption. As an example, a national real income growth of 5% per head per year is a high target; the elasticity of food energy consumption, as a national average for developing countries, is around 0.2-0.4 (*16*); for low-income groups it may be higher, of the order of 0.5-0.6. As another example, if the projected increase in income generated by an investment project were around 10% per head per year, this would give up to 6% food consumption increase. Thus a 3-6% increase in food consumption per head per year would be a considerable achievement. With such figures, a household consuming 80% of requirement would on average reach 100% in 5-10 years, and the prevalence of malnutrition could be measurably reduced over this period. Thus, under circumstances of high income growth, it would be reasonable to expect measurable changes in nutritional status over say 5-10 years; equally in most other circumstances little change would be expected (taken from Mason, *17*).

In many development projects, one concern in setting objectives is with economic calculations to assess the project's viability in the above terms. Thus, a possible basis for specifying nutritional targets may be available from economic data; for example, income targets might in theory be usable for projecting food consumption effects. One attempt to develop methods of assessing in advance a programme's nutritional impact has been made by the World Bank, through programme effects on output, price, income, and other influences on the consumption of households with malnourished members. The quantification of these factors requires that a number of parameters, such as income and price elasticities, be estimated, which is normally a difficult undertaking. Hence, it may still be some time before this or some similar framework becomes fully operational. None the less, such an approach may in the future provide a way of quantifying expected nutritional outcome, at least in terms of energy consumption. A second approach, used by FAO (*18*), stops at the point of attempting to predict broad trends in nutritional status (improvement, no change, deterioration), because of the difficulty in projecting changes in energy intakes.[1]

Thus, there is only a sketchy methodological basis at present for setting quantified nutritional objectives via economic effects. However, an obvious starting-point in evaluation of nutritional effects is within programmes in which likely nutritional effects have at least been considered in the planning stage.

Setting adequacy criteria for outcome indicators

Outcome objectives could be set in several ways, ranging from the best possible outcome (i.e., elimination of the problem), through the outcome reasonably to be expected if the programme is satisfactorily carried out, to a minimum acceptable outcome. The last of these – which can be a different level depending on whether it is a short- or long-term programme – establishes the criterion for adequacy of the outcome. Any outcome less than this indicates the

---

[1] *Report on review discussions of FAO methods for introducing nutritional considerations into agricultural and rural development projects, held in FAO, Rome 19-21 February 1980.* Rome, Food and Agriculture Organization of the United Nations, 1980 (mimeographed document).

need for modification of the current procedures or, possibly, discontinuation of the programme. (Further evaluation may be required to determine the causes of the apparent failure.)

Methods of cost-effectiveness analysis are in fact used, explicitly or implicitly, in determining the minimum, the decision often being based only on subjective judgement – i.e., *some* level of effect is decided to be just worth the cost. For example, the number of cases of malnutrition to be prevented (or rehabilitated) per unit of expenditure could be estimated. It has not been possible to establish consistent results on the basis of such costs and effects. However, as an example we have calculated from some of the available data on supplementary feeding programmes (including certain of those reviewed by Gwatkin et al., *11*) that typical expenditure may be around US$ 10–20 per child recipient per year, with a cost of very roughly US$ 50–200 per child rehabilitated.

In any event, this process must lead to a planning decision on the trend over time of values of the outcome indicator defining the minimum acceptable result of the programme. Evaluating the adequacy of outcome could then be envisaged as plotting values of the outcome indicator on a graph of this trend. A hypothetical example is shown in Fig. 5.2. Here, a minimum adequacy level has been specified as a decrease in the prevalence of malnutrition from 30% to 20% over six years. At year 2, the outcome was inadequate, which led to tightening up of the management procedures; thereafter the outcome was considered adequate on annual evaluation.

The considered population depends on how the objectives were set. It can be the recipients, in which case allowance must also be made for deviation from targeting objectives. Frequently, the criteria for admission to a programme are the same as the outcome indicators. For example, the admission criterion could be a weight-for-age less than 80% of standard on screening, weight gain being then used as the measure of outcome. In this case, regression to the mean – i.e., the improvement that would occur without the programme due to selection of an extreme group – is an important confounding factor (see ref. *19*). This can only be allowed for if estimates of the spontaneous rate of improvement are available. While the gross outcome does not take this confounding into account, the rate of recovery that would anyway be expected without the programme must be considered when setting adequacy criteria.

One way of making allowance for deviation from the targeting objectives is by estimating the outcome for the target population as the criterion for adequacy. This can only be done from data on recipients, assuming that the prevalence for non-recipients is unchanged. Otherwise, data on outcome indicators for non-recipients are needed. Again, consideration of regression to the mean is needed if the targeting criteria involve screening (i.e., the targeted and the needy are the same).

Finally, the outcome for the population as a whole could be the criterion of adequacy. This normally requires data on non-recipients, which are not usually obtainable through programme contacts but in most cases require survey work.

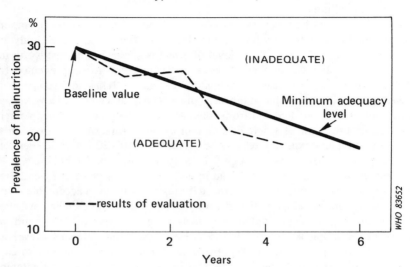

Fig. 5.2. Evaluating outcome adequacy:
a hypothetical example [a]

[a] The population to which the prevalence refers should be specified, i.e., recipients, target group, needy, whole population (see text).

Common nutritional outcome indicators for protein-energy malnutrition

The nutritional outcome indicators used for evaluation are much the same as those discussed in Chapter 4. These are in line with the health status indicators defined for evaluation of health programmes (*1*, pp. 21-22).

For a recent review of experience in using such indicators for evaluation of feeding programmes, we drew up a table listing the known responsiveness of such indicators and a second table of more qualitative available experience (*2*, Tables 10 and 11). Anthropometric indicators (weight, height, and age) in children were found to be consistently the most responsive in a field (as opposed to a hospital) setting. More qualitative experience could be summarized as shown in Table 5.4 (adapted from Table 10 in the review quoted above).

The use of several different anthropometric indicators for programme evaluation has been reviewed by Habicht & Butz *(9)*. They concluded that both height and weight are sensitive to nutrition intervention programmes, especially if measured longitudinally in the same children. Height increments were found to be more sensitive than weight increments in the sense of producing greater statistical significance.

Infant and child mortality rates have also been used to assess outcome (e.g., by Gwatkin et al., *11*). These are clearly of fundamental interest, but are difficult to collect accurately except when there is individual contact and careful follow-up of project participants. Hence they are more suitable for pilot programmes. In health programmes particularly, assessment of disease prevalences (cases at one point in time) and incidences (numbers of new cases per unit of time) are often used with varying success. These data are of interest both in medical care and in preventive and environmental health programmes. Here again, results are easier to get when there is individual contact. From the studies reviewed by Habicht & Butz *(9)*, the conclusion was that mortality and morbidity rates did not provide sensitive indicators of changes in nutrition, i.e., that the effects of intervention were not easily detected by measuring these variables. The projects reviewed by Gwatkin et al. *(11)* led these authors to value mortality rates more highly as indicators, when health care is included in the interventions.

Other outcome indicators that could be more widely used in this context in the future, and that have been discussed in Chapter 4, are prevalence of low birth weight and height of children at school entry. For further discussion of the characteristics of nutritional status indicators see Habicht *(20)*.

Organization

The organization of ongoing evaluation obviously depends on the type of programme involved, the way the management structure is set up, and the reasons for the evaluation. In all cases, the organization for ongoing evaluation must be established with clear links to those making the management decisions on the programme for which the evaluation is being made – preferably as an integral part of the management structure.

Many regular government programmes (e.g., health services) aim at national coverage. Some decision-making may be decentralized, and sometimes the capacity to evaluate may exist at these decentralized levels. For certain more specific programmes – e.g., feeding programmes – governments may decide as a political measure that a programme should reach the entire population in the country or all individuals within a certain demographic group (e.g., school lunches will be served to all children in all schools of the country). Again, some decentralized decision-making may be possible and the evaluation capacity has to be established accordingly. On the other hand, a government with few economic resources may decide, for example, to implement a supplementary feeding programme targeted to undernourished preschool children in the most deprived region of the country: this type of programme is not only targeted by region but also by screening for selection of beneficiaries. Evaluation here is clearly specific to the region.

Table 5.4. Outcome indicators for evaluation in relation to selected programmes and objectives [a]

Programme type	Objectives	Indicators	
		A. Widely used and recommended for evaluation	B. Less often used—mainly for research studies
1. Preschool child programmes	(a) Reduce protein-energy malnutrition	A. Wt and ht changes Ht/age, wt/age, wt/ht	B. Clinical signs Dietary intake Limb circumferences and skinfolds
	(b) Reduce morbidity	A/B Prevalence of diseases No. of episodes Duration longitudinally	
	(c) Reduce infant and child mortality		B. Infant and child mortality rates
2. School feeding programmes	(a) Improve nutritional status	A. Heights and weights longitudinally	B. Other anthropometric and biochemical tests
	(b) Improve school enrolment and attendance	A. Records of enrolment and attendance	
	(c) Improve school performance		B. School performance tests
	(d) Income transfer; increased food intake		B. Consumption, income, expenditure
3. Food for work programmes	(a) Increase productivity		B. Physical activity, energy expenditure
	(b) Increase income and/or food consumption	A/B Household surveys of expenditure	
4. Relief in emergencies	(a) Rehabilitation: children	A. Anthropometry; clinical signs	
	(b) Rehabilitation: adults	A. Weight gain	
5. Supplementary feeding for mothers	Reduce: risks at birth, low birth weight, subsequent infant mortality	A. Weight gain during pregnancy; birth weight	B. Perinatal and/or infant mortality rates

[a] Source: adapted from Table 10 in ref. 2.

Rural development programmes are likely to be confined to certain areas, and moreover often have a distinct management structure within, or sometimes separate from, the government agencies involved. Here again there is a clear place for ongoing evaluation within programme management.

Deciding responsibilities

In organizing ongoing evaluation for programme management, certain responsibilities have to be agreed and clearly defined at the outset:
– Who is responsible for *decisions* concerning the results of the evaluation, and for *initiating* the evaluation in the first place?
– Who is responsible for *managing the evaluation?*
– Who is responsible for *data collection, processing and analysis?*

Those responsible for decisions are clearly the programme management, generally with guidance from a central policy body and/or donors. However, the management itself may not always take the initiative for implementing evaluation – even if this is designed into the programme. In fact, initiatives for programme evaluation usually come from higher levels in the planning structure – administrators and funders. None the less, it is clear, as pointed out in ref. *1* (page 15), that those responsible for decisions should be responsible also for the evaluation leading to those decisions.

The first objective should be to improve the management of the programme and it is to this purpose that the methods discussed here are suited. Often, there are further objectives – to determine whether or not to expand the programme, or even whether to initiate similar programmes elsewhere. It should be kept in mind and made explicit, however, that the limited but important use of adequacy evaluation is primarily as a means of improving the programme itself. For other purposes – to assess net outcome or impact, or to decide whether to expand a programme in the same area or, still more, in a dissimilar area – additional data and analysis are usually required and these requirements are beyond the scope of adequacy evaluation. Attention has already been drawn to this limitation on p. 142, but it merits re-emphasizing.

Different types of institutional arrangement may be needed, depending upon the source of information to be used, for example when:
– data are generated routinely by the programme; in this case outcome data are usually restricted to programme contacts;
– data are generated by other sources, e.g., from administrative sources, possibly as part of a national nutritional surveillance system;
– data are generated through special purpose surveys (outside or inside the programme).

The institutional arrangements must also include assignment of responsibilities for data analysis and interpretation of results.

Organization of data collection

The organization of data collection and analysis discussed in Chapter 3 is similar in principle to that for adequacy evaluation of nutritional effects of programmes. The major differences include the following:

(*a*) The population to be monitored will generally be smaller, and a higher sampling rate (either a random sample, or drawn from existing data sources such as clinics) will be needed; disaggregation of national data to refer to a programme area is often not feasible because of sample size limitations.

(*b*) Process data must be included.

(*c*) Data from programme contacts may be available (e.g., from children receiving food supplements, farmers visited by extension workers).

(*d*) The linkage to decision-making should be much closer in relation to specific programmes.

Data from programme contacts

The distinction has been made between data on recipients and on the population as a whole. The acquisition of data from direct contacts can be both process (on delivery) and, with suitable organization, outcome (e.g., weights of children). Baseline data can be used to complement programme-obtained data.

In many programmes it may be easier to obtain data on programme recipients than on the population as a whole. Usually, however, the objective is to follow changes in gross outcome for the planned target group (which may not be the same as recipients in practice); these can be represented by points on the graph in Fig. 5.2. When the delivery of the programme succeeds in reaching all the target population, and only the target population, data on recipients are equivalent to data on the target group. When recipients are not exactly the same as the target group, outcome for the target group can still be estimated if an assumption can be made that there has been no change among non-recipients.

When measurements are obtained routinely as part of the programme, e.g., by weighing children in a maternal and child health programme, the main need is to gather these data just as data are gathered from other administrative sources, as discussed in Chapter 4. Even if measurements are not routinely obtained, but there is contact, e.g., through household visits, it may be feasible for the programme staff to collect data periodically on a sample, e.g., by interview or weighing of children.

Routine data from administrative sources

Methods of data collection from clinics, schools, local government, etc., have been reviewed in Chapter 4. The same procedures apply in general to using these data for adequacy evaluations of projects. Two additions are needed, which are likely to be more feasible and useful when linked to a particular programme than when not so linked. The first concerns the possibility of using variables to control for changing extent of services. The second relates to the organization of data collection.

One problem with routine data in this case – we will take clinic data as an illustration – is not so much that their absolute relation to the overall population is unknown as that the interpretation of *changes* detected in a clinic-attending population is confounded by possible changes in the clinic's coverage. Periodic representative surveys are one solution, but are costly. Another solution worth trying would be to estimate changes in coverage itself in some way. For example, recording and comparing estimates of the distance travelled to the clinic would allow changes in coverage to be assessed.

The organization of data collection to maintain a flow of reliable data from routine sources is also fundamental. It applies to all forms of surveillance, but is included here since it is reckoned more likely that the resources needed to tackle it could be made available in a programme context, at least to begin with. Much has been said (e.g., ref. *21*) about the need to ensure two-way information flows, one purpose of which is to motivate data collectors to continue. There is little experience of two-way flows, and less evidence that it is effective in maintaining data collection. It may be more realistic to assume that, for instance, clinic personnel will collect and record information (such as diagnosis) for their own purposes but will have little enthusiasm for copying, collating, and passing this information on. It is, after all, not their job. An alternative solution is to employ staff specifically to do this – indeed this is what is done in some developed countries (e.g., the USA). Not so many people would be needed, if the recorded information were sampled. It might be envisaged that an enumerator could get adequate data by visiting any particular clinic once a month. The enumerator could extract the data from a sample of existing records (e.g., patients' notes) if these are kept at the clinic. If not, the enumerator would have to gather data on the sample of patients attending the clinic on that particular day. This system would at least assure a regular flow of data of relatively consistent reliability. It would also impose record sampling at the source of data.

Data from community weighing

The use of community weighing programmes has also been discussed in Chapter 4. The weighing programme in the Philippines, carried out once or twice yearly, is an example. Stations are set up village by village, with the aim of weighing all children over a period of about three days. The results (weights and ages) are reported by the village to the municipality (typically 20 to 30 per municipality). The primary use is for the village-level targeting of the Philippine nutrition programme, as planned by the municipal nutrition committee. Comparison of the results, by village and year, could evidently give indicators of programme adequacy. The difficulty is that coverage of the population to be weighed is very variable and can be well below 50% of the preschool population. None the less, elements of a local evaluation system do exist. Such data could permit estimates as to whether rates of change in malnutrition were adequate. With information on programme delivery, they could also assess targeting.

Special purpose surveys

Two types of survey have been used. First, a census of heights of schoolchildren has been carried out in Costa Rica and the Philippines. Second, small-scale surveys have been carried out for programme design, repetition of which would give the needed information for evaluation. Four such surveys were recently carried out with FAO assistance, specifically designed to provide minimal information on nutritional conditions in a project area *(22)*. They are thus possible examples of the type of survey that could be repeated in surveillance, and are described briefly for this purpose.

These surveys were expected to provide, as primary outputs, selected indicators of nutritional conditions and related factors, disaggregated by socioeconomic group. Three types of data were collected: characteristics by area and by household, and indicators of outcome.[1] The surveys typically covered 250 to 1000 households in project areas with population of 20 000 to 300 000. The time required for the surveys from design to presentation of descriptive results was 4–6 months. The cost was of the order of US$ 50 000 per survey.

The suitability of surveys such as these, regularly repeated for evaluation purposes, depends first, on whether they will produce the right data, and second, on whether they can be repeated. The data produced are suitable for assessing changes in certain aspects of nutrition and living levels. The indicators selected are those that are objectively measurable (e.g., child's weight), easy to observe (e.g., type of housing, sanitation facilities), or needing the minimum of recall (e.g., current sickness/health). Feasibility of repetition is more complex. It depends on administrative capacity, personnel available, funds, and so on. It is clear that the financial cost of such surveys falls within the allocations made in, for example, many development programmes (see ref. *4*). The organizational needs are similar to those of other surveys. Personnel requirements are also similar, since it has turned out to be no more difficult to train enumerators for these nutritional indicator surveys than for other purposes. Often such data can be collected as part of broader-purpose surveys undertaken for more general project evaluation, as discussed below.

---

[1] For example, see: MASON, J.B. *Case-study for FAO on introducing nutrition considerations into development project planning – Haiti*. Ithaca, NY, Cornell University, 1980 (mimeographed document).

Nutrition measurements within programme evaluation surveys

It may be a more practical proposition in many circumstances to include nutrition measurements in other surveys, rather than to set up surveys primarily for nutrition measurements. This is equivalent to the "nutrition module" concept discussed in Chapter 4, and details will not be repeated here. The advantages of incorporating nutrition measurements in another survey are obvious. Not only are resources easier to come by, but many other aspects of survey procedures – e.g., sampling, hiring and training enumerators, logistics – will already be partially taken care of.

Examples

In practice, evaluations of many operational programmes disregard most confounding variables and the organizers are content to establish the adequacy of the programme even if this compromise is not made explicit. Most available reports, such as those quoted earlier in this chapter, are from pilot rather than routine programmes. Regular evaluation of operational programmes is not common or even frequently written up. However, two examples, given below, are illuminating. A programme targeted by screening is given first and a non-target programme next. These approximate to the ideas of adequacy evaluation. Finally, we discuss adequacy evaluation in the context of the effects of development programmes.

Example 1 – Targeted maternal and child health programme (Philippines)

A targeted maternal and child health programme, designed to feed over 1.1 million preschool children between the ages of 6 and 72 months during a four-year period, as well as 100 000 pregnant and lactating women, was begun in 1972 in the Philippines. Beneficiaries of the programme were identified by a house-to-house weighing survey. Children 75% of standard weight-for-age or less were eligible, as were all pregnant and lactating women. Children were weighed each month and remained in the programme until their weights exceeded 75% standard weight-for-age. The programme was carried out in feeding centres. One centre was intended to provide food for 150-175 children and 40-50 mothers, equivalent to an additional daily ration of 1.8 MJ (430 kcal) and 20 g protein per person. Mothers of malnourished children and pregnant and lactating women also received education in health and nutrition and demonstrations in the preparation of the distributed food.

The nutritionists in charge of each centre completed the information in Table 5.5 each month for each child. Collating these data provided information on the number of beneficiaries (both children and mothers). Participation was compared with the previously set monthly targets. Collating results from the

Table 5.5. Targeted maternal and child health programme: nutrition weight record (Philippines) [a]

Health region _____   Centre No. _____

Province _____   Barrio _____
                                   (or mothercraft class No.)
Municipality _____

Barrio _____   Date class began _____

                                 Supervisor _____

Name of recipient _____ Sex ____ Birth date _____

Age in months _____   Age group _____
(At initial food issue)

Time of weighing	Date	Weight	% standard weight	Nutrition level	Weight gain	% of standard gain	Gain level	Comments
Initial								
Follow-up								

Family history:
How many living children do you have _____ No. dead _____
                                                (including fetal deaths)

How many children older _____

How many children younger _____ Months older _____

Birth date of next youngest child _____ Months younger _____

Weight of child at birth _____ Length of child at birth _____

[a] Source: Caedo, M. & Engel, R.W. *The mothercraft concept applied to Southeast Asia,* 1973 (mimeographed document).

individual weight records (Table 5.5) also permitted monthly reporting of the progress of each child.

Periodic evaluation of the gross outcome of the project was made by comparing the number of rehabilitated children with yearly targets (see Table 5.6). For example, by July 1975, 468 000 children were to have been rehabilitated.

Certain results of monitoring the weights of participating children in the programme are shown in Table 5.7 Improvements in weight-for-age are shown three months after enrolment and again six months after. Enrolment of children was scheduled to last 18–24 months. If the group of children continued to gain weight by one percentage point every three months, children 2 years of age and

Table 5.6. Number of children rehabilitated (thousands) [a,b]

Month	Fiscal year					
	1972	1973	1974	1975	1976	1977
July		44	206	468	756	978
August		52	226	492	780	990
September		60	246	516	804	1 002
October	2	71	267	540	825	1 011
November	4	82	288	564	846	1 020
December	6	93	309	588	867	1 029
January	10	107	331	612	885	
February	14	121	353	636	903	
March	18	135	375	660	921	
April	24	152	398	684	936	
May	39	169	421	708	951	
June	36	189	444	732	966	

[a] Source: Caido & Engel, 1973 (see Table 5.5).
[b] These figures are targets not achievements.

Table 5.7. Child weight responses in a targeted maternal
and child health programme:
summary of 8 classes, 1971-1972 [a,b]

Age range (months)	Body weight as % of standard		
	Initial or base line	After 3 months	After 6 months
6–13	71.4	73.0	74.3
24–71	73.4	74.4	75.3
All ages	72.8	73.9	74.9

[a] Source: Caedo & Engel, 1973 (see Table 5.5).
[b] These classes (n = 542) were operated by Catholic relief service nutritionists. Participants were families residing in the low-income and squatter resettlements of Greater Manila, Philippines.

older would have reached the goal of 80% of standard at the end of 24 months, while the younger children would have been very close to this goal.

The above is an example of a large-scale feeding programme in which monitoring and evaluation for adequacy were greatly simplified. The only data recorded were participation and weight gains. No control group was used, and the evaluation method did not endeavour to show cause and effect. The target group was carefully identified, as were expected participation rates and weight gains over a specified time period. This type of approach to monitoring and evaluation gives the programme manager useful information on whether or not the programme is proceeding smoothly. At the same time, the demands of data collection and reporting can be met by the field staff.

Example 2 – Vitamin A programmes in Central America and Panama

National nutrition surveys conducted by the Institute of Nutrition of Central America and Panama (INCAP) in 1965-1967 *(23)* identified vitamin A deficiency as one of the major nutritional problems affecting the population of Central America and Panama. The nutritional indicators used to make that assertion were estimates of family and child intake of vitamin A sources, clinical symptoms of deficiency, and prevalence of low and deficient levels of serum retinol (less than 0.7 µmol/l). INCAP conducted extensive laboratory research to find a chemical product that could be added to a food widely consumed by target populations (poor rural families) suffering from vitamin A deficiency, and found that retinol palmitate could be added to common sugar *(24)*. Analysis of available food consumption surveys showed that sugar was a suitable vehicle for delivering vitamin A to poor rural families, as it was widely used and consumed in quantities that allow for a reasonable fortification level (15 µg of retinol per gram of sugar). Problems of transferring research results to a national programme were overcome in 1972, and in 1975 Costa Rica and Guatemala began nation-wide fortification of sugar with vitamin A.

INCAP conducted evaluations of the vitamin A programme among poor rural families of Guatemala from 1975 to 1978, using before-and-after measurements as well as control groups receiving unfortified sugar. Baseline and subsequent periodic surveys were undertaken to obtain data on total food consumption and retinol content in human milk, to carry out clinical examinations, and to ascertain levels of serum retinol in children and other age-groups. Samples of sugar sold in the local shops and markets were collected to determine whether there was an impact on vitamin A status as a result of the intervention, whether sugar was really being fortified, and whether the fortified sugar was reaching poor children. The results are given in Table 5.8. The percentage of children with serum retinol levels below 0.7 µmol/l (20 µg/100 ml) dropped from 21.5% before the programme to 9.2% after two years of intervention.

In Costa Rica, data available for 1978 and comparisons of serum retinol levels of children in 1966 and in 1979 (5 years after fortification started in 1975) demonstrated a dramatic improvement in the percentage of children with deficient or low levels of serum retinol (32.5% in 1966 and 2.3% in 1978). By comparison, in El Salvador, where no vitamin A programme was carried out, a drop in percentage of children with deficient and low levels of retinol from 1966 to 1976 was also identified (50.0% in 1966 and 33.3% in 1976), although it was not as large as those in Guatemala and Costa Rica.[1] The improvement in Costa Rica was considered to be satisfactory, and was in practice, probably reasonably, attributed at least in part to the fortification programme on the basis of findings such as these. The more important conclusion for management,

---

[1] VALVERDE, V. ET AL. *Overview of nutritional status in the Western Hemisphere: Central America and Panama.* Paper read at the Western Hemisphere Nutrition Congress VI, 10-14 August 1980 in Los Angeles, CA, USA, 1980 (unpublished document).

however, was that vitamin A deficiency was decreasing dramatically (whether or not this could be attributed to the programme). Pending more extensive evaluation, it was reasonable to continue the programme.

Table 5.8. Number and percentage of preschool children with different serum retinol levels, Guatemala, 1975-1977 [a]

Survey period	Total No. of cases	Serum retinol level (µg/100 ml) [b]							
		<10		10-19		20-29		≥30	
		No.	(%)	No.	(%)	No.	(%)	No.	(%)
Oct-Nov 1975	549	18	(3.3)[c]	100	(18.2)	189	(34.4)	242	(44.1)
Apr-May 1976	583	6	(1.0)	77	(13.1)	205	(35.5)	295	(50.4)
Oct-Nov 1976	645	2	(0.3)	31	(4.8)	165	(25.6)	447	(69.3)
Apr-May 1977	674	6	(0.9)	69	(10.2)	189	(28.0)	410	(60.9)
Oct-Nov 1977	721	2	(0.3)	64	(8.9)	260	(36.1)	395	(54.6)

[a] Source: Arroyave et al. (24), p. 30.
[b] 1 µg/100 ml = 0.035 µmol/l.
[c] Figures in parentheses = percentage of cases.

Experience in monitoring and evaluation of development programmes

Experience in the monitoring and evaluation of development programmes is perhaps more relevant to adequacy evaluation than many of the studies of health/nutrition projects, which have usually been of a research nature. These monitoring and evaluation systems are intended to provide information internal to the programmes and relevant to management decisions. What is emphasized is process monitoring and, in practice, the obtaining of data on gross outcome rather than net impact. It is instructive to review briefly both the similarities and differences between project monitoring and evaluation, on the one hand, and nutritional surveillance, on the other. There are many parallels in the problems faced, in their identification, approaches to solving them, objectives, and so on. This means not only that those concerned with surveillance can learn from these parallel experiences and deliberations, but also that advances in surveillance may find a use in the monitoring and evaluation of development programmes. The differences have important implications too, the most obvious of which is the much greater extent of these activities and the vastly greater resources applied, primarily by donor agencies. For example, the World Bank review of monitoring and evaluation of projects in East Africa in 1979 (4) gives a figure of 12.8 million dollars for monitoring and evaluation of 28 projects with a budget for this averaging US$ 460 000 each. This is about 0.5 to 5% of total project costs. Similar figures were derived from a review of projects in East Asia.[1] Indeed, the level of resource commitment to monitoring and evaluation of large-scale investment projects rivals that of entire national statistical operations.

The present status of project monitoring and evaluation can be conveniently traced by reference to recent workshops and publications on the subject. The World Bank held three regional workshops between 1977 and 1979, in East Africa, East Asia, and Latin America *(4)*,[1] and the Organization for Economic Cooperation and Development (OECD) sponsored a meeting in 1977 and has issued a number of useful publications *(6, 25, 26)*.

One of the OECD books *(26*, pp. 13-14) states:

"A review of the state of the art suggests, whether looking at management information systems in general or at specific components (measurements, social indicators, evaluation, monitoring), the following conclusions: there exists a general agreement on what should be done; there exists very little information on how to do it in a specific project setting... a clear shift in concerns can be observed: increasingly, emphasis is laid upon the applicability of information systems; concern has shifted away from monitoring/evaluation techniques to the management's use of evaluation results... from how to measure and analyse to what to measure and how to present the information to management."

The parallel with the methods discussed in this chapter is clear.

There is still a substantial gap between design and implementation; between indicators proposed and those actually collected. The late 1970s saw the compilation of many lists of indicators for monitoring development (e.g., ref. *27-31)*. Partly because of the need to satisfy multidisciplinary interests, the lists were extensive and often failed to distinguish data types in terms of collection requirements. Thus, for example, crop yields and production by farm type and disaggregated income and food consumption data were widely proposed. This also led to considerable complexity in design, on the occasions when these lists were translated into project proposals. For example, one proposal for systems for monitoring and evaluating nutritional interventions *(32)* lists more than 50 "objectively verifiable indicators", including energy intakes, areas planted, etc., with much numerical detail as to intended targets. Similarly, the document on monitoring rural development *(29)* lists several hundred indicators.

Difficulties in implementing such complex schemes have led to simplification in concepts. The World Bank has proposed a very much more limited list of outcome indicators, including nutritional status *(33*, p. 43-45). These authors conclude

"nutritional status merits consideration as a proxy composite indicator for health and food consumption... anthropometric indicators are proxies for the nutritional status of the child population and these, in turn, are used as proxies for reflecting the general levels of health and food consumption of the population under study. The great advantages of anthropometric indicators lies in the ease of collection of the necessary data on large samples and their reasonable sensitivity to

---

[1] DEBOECK, G. & NG, R. *Monitoring rural development in East Asia*. Washington, DC, World Bank, 1980 (draft World Bank Working Paper).

change in the underlying variables of interest. Clearly, they do not mirror the population's specific health problems, but as indicators ... of the quality of life ... [they] can be strongly recommended for more general evaluation purposes."

Other indicators recommended for monitoring and evaluation of agricultural and rural development projects in this publication are also similar to those used in nutritional surveillance: for example, shelter as measured by the quality of housing; distance from, or time to reach, potable water; use of clinics. Further, the classifying information suggested is also similar (*33*, p. 45): geographical location and community characteristics; demographic characteristics; farm size and type; and main economic activities or occupation.

Most of the examples of monitoring and evaluation of development programmes rely both on administrative reporting and sample surveys for process data; and, where outcome data are to be collected, primarily on sample surveys for these. A summary of 19 programmes, taken from one of the World Bank workshops, is given in Table 5.9. From this it can be seen that data collection and analysis always relate to project inputs and ouputs, derived substantially from project reports; and to selected project effects, obtained usually by sample survey. The only common outcome variable in this review was income, usually to be obtained by sample survey. It seems that monitoring develops from process to effects, and that while most projects aim to gain outcome data, this is not always achieved.

Table 5.9. Analysis of case-studies of monitoring and evaluation of development programmes in East Asia: planned and implemented methods of data collection on process, effects (e.g., crop yields) and outcome (e.g., income) [a]

Data collection method	Process		Effects		Outcome	
	Planned	Done	Planned	Done	Planned	Done
Reporting only	6	5	3	2	2	1
Sample survey only	5	2	6	3	4	0
Both	8	3	7	0	6	0
Total	19	10	16	5	12	1

[a] Source: extracted from Deboeck & Ng, 1980 (see footnote, p. 172).

Data processing and analysis seem to be almost universal problems in monitoring and evaluation of effects and impact. Requirements are underestimated, resources inadequate (in absolute terms and compared with those put into data collection), and long delays are the general rule. This seems to apply less to process data, presumably since this is derived more from project reporting, which requires less analysis.

This experience urges caution in looking at ways in which nutritional surveillance can contribute to evaluation, but it also helps to explain and put in context the rather slow progress in the evaluation aspects of surveillance. The starting-point should be the same as that for monitoring and evaluation of development programmes quoted earlier: applicability of systems; use of results; and what to measure and how to present information usefully. It is clear that nutritional surveillance is on the same track as other evaluation methods, and may have a particular role to play in assisting in the use of anthropometric and health data, for example as recommended for more general monitoring by Casley & Lury *(33)*. It may also help in the development of methods for obtaining such data, both within sample surveys and from administrative sources, particularly clinics.

REFERENCES

1. *Health programme evaluation. Guiding principles for its application to the managerial process for national health development*. Geneva, World Health Organization, 1981 ("Health for All" Series, No. 6).
2. HABICHT, J.-P. ET AL. Basic concepts for design of evaluations during program implementation. In: Sahn, D. E. et al., ed. *Methods for evaluating the impact of food and nutrition programs*. Tokyo, United Nations University (in press).
3. MASON, J. B. & HABICHT, J.-P. Stages of evaluation of on-going programs. In: Sahn, D. E. et al., ed. *Methods of evaluating the impact of food and nutrition programs*. Tokyo, United Nations University (in press).
4. DEBOECK, G. & KINSEY, B. *Managing information for rural development: Lessons from Eastern Africa*. Washington, DC, World Bank, 1980 (World Bank Staff Working Paper, No. 379).
5. SAHN, D. E. & PESTRONK, R. M. *A review of issues in nutrition program evaluation*. Washington, DC, US Agency for International Development, 1981 (AID Program Evaluation Discussion Paper, No. 10).
6. FREEMAN, H. E. ET AL. *Evaluating social projects in developing countries*. Paris, Organization for Economic Cooperation and Development, 1979.
7. CAMPBELL, D. T. & STANLEY, J. C. *Experimental and quasi-experimental designs for research*. Chicago, Rand McNally, 1966.
8. COOK, T. D. & CAMPBELL, D. T. *Quasi-experimentation*. Boston, Houghton Mifflin, 1979.
9. HABICHT, J.-P. & BUTZ, W. P. Measurement of health and nutrition effects of large-scale nutrition intervention projects. In: Klein, R. E. et al., ed. *Evaluating the impact of nutrition and health programs*. New York, Plenum Press, 1979.
10. BEATON, G. H. & GHASSEMI, H. Supplementary feeding programs for young children in developing countries. *American journal of clinical nutrition*, **35**: 864-916 (1982).
11. GWATKIN, D. R. ET AL. *Can health and nutrition interventions make a difference?* Washington, DC, Overseas Development Council, 1980 (ODC Monograph, No. 13).
12. DRAKE, W. D. ET AL. *Final report: Analysis of community-level nutrition programs. Project analysis of community-level nutrition programs*, vol. 1. Washington, DC, US Agency for International Development, 1980.
13. AUSTIN, J. E. & ZEITLIN, M. F. *Nutrition intervention in developing countries*. Cambridge, MA, Oelgeschlager, Gunn & Hain, 1981.

14. HABICHT, J.-P. Specifications of a national nutrition information system. In: Inoue, G. & Yoshimura, H., ed. *Effects of alterations of dietary patterns and food habits on health*. Tokyo, Japanese Malnutrition Panel of US-Japan Cooperative Medical Sciences Program, 1979.

15. PYLE, D. F. Nutrition interventions: Problems associated with expanding pilot/demonstration projects into national level programs. In: Harper, A. E. & Davis, G. K. *Progress in clinical and biological research*, vol. 77 - Nutrition in health and disease and international development. *Symposia from XIIth International Congress of Nutrition*. New York, Alan R. Liss Inc., 1981, pp. 575-584.

16. *Agricultural commodity projection, 1970-1980*, vol. II. Rome, Food and Agriculture Organization of the United Nations, 1971 (Publication CCP 71/20).

17. MASON, J. B. Agricultural and economic components of nutritional surveillance. *Food and nutrition*, **4**: 21-26 (1978).

18. *Nutrition in agriculture. Fifth session of the Committee on Agriculture*. Rome, Food and Agriculture Organization of the United Nations, 1979 (Publication COAG 7916).

19. DAVIS, C. E. The effect of regression to the mean in epidemiologic and clinical studies. *American journal of epidemiology*, **104**: 493-498 (1976).

20. HABICHT, J.-P. Some characteristics of indicators of nutritional status for use in screening and surveillance. *American journal of clinical nutrition*, **33**: 531-535 (1980).

21. WHO Technical Report Series, No. 593, 1976 *(Methodology of nutritional surveillance. Report of a Joint FAO/UNICEF/WHO Expert Committee)*.

22. *Introducing nutrition in agriculture and rural development*. Rome, Food and Agriculture Organization of the United Nations, 1980 (Publication COAG 81/6).

23. INCAP/INTERDEPARTMENTAL COMMITTEE ON NUTRITION FOR NATIONAL DEVELOPMENT. *Nutritional evaluation of the population of Central America and Panama, 1965-1967*. Washington, DC, US Department of Health, Education, and Welfare, 1971 (US DHEW Publication No. (HSM) 72-8120).

24. ARROYAVE, G. ET AL. *Evaluation of sugar fortification with vitamin A at the national level*. Washington, DC, Pan American Health Organization, 1979 (Scientific Publication 384).

25. IMBODEN, N. *A management approach to project appraisal and evaluation, with special reference to non-directly productive projects*. Paris, Organization for Economic Development and Cooperation, 1978.

26. IMBODEN, N. *Managing information for rural development projects*. Paris, Organization for Economic Development and Cooperation, 1980.

27. BASTER, N. *Social indicators and social statistics in context to FAO's concerns*. Rome, Food and Agriculture Organization of the United Nations, 1978.

28. DEBOECK, G. J. *Systems for monitoring and evaluating nutritional interventions*. Washington, DC, World Bank, 1978.

29. WEISEL, P. F. & MICKELWAIT, D. R. *Designing rural development projects: an approach*. Washington, DC, Development Alternatives, Inc., 1978.

30. UNITED NATIONS. DEPARTMENT OF INTERNATIONAL ECONOMIC AND SOCIAL AFFAIRS. STATISTICAL OFFICE. *The National Household Survey Capability Programme. Prospectus*. New York, United Nations, 1980 (DP/UN/INT-79-020/1), Annex III.

31. *World Conference on Agrarian Reform and Rural Development (WCAARD) Report. Rome, 12-20 July 1979*. Rome, Food and Agriculture Organization of the United Nations, 1979, p. 6, section D.

32. CERNEA, M. M. & TEPPING, B. J. *A system for monitoring and evaluating agricultural extension projects*. Washington, DC, World Bank, 1977 (World Bank Staff Working Paper No. 272).

33. CASLEY, D. J. & LURY, D. A. *A handbook on monitoring and evaluation of agricultural and rural development projects*. Washington, DC, World Bank, 1981.

CHAPTER 6

Timely warning and intervention programmes

Summary

Timely warning and intervention programmes can be designed to prevent acute food shortages. They involve predetermined interventions and the necessary data to trigger them. This applies both to food shortages of famine proportions and to severe localized seasonal shortages. Timely warning and intervention programmes are worth considering when there is a risk of acute food shortage (often due to drought), when the resources to prevent or relieve the shortage are potentially available, and when lack of information is a constraint.

Timely warning means at the right time so that intervention can be initiated to prevent seriously declining food consumption. Operationally, three time-periods need to be considered: the lag due to data flow; the delay in mobilizing the intervention; and the time for the intervention to have a positive or stabilizing effect on food consumption. The interventions themselves may tackle basic causes of the problem (e.g., by seed or pesticide distribution), or intermediate causes (e.g., by income support); if these fail, relief measures may be needed. Finally, the long-run solution is to prevent vulnerability to food shortage itself. Interventions can be graded to deal successfully with these basic and intermediate causes. Decisions on different interventions require different indicators, referred to as early, concurrent, and later. Administrative data may give a "yellow light" early warning, leading to more focused analysis or data collection for concurrent indicators. The concept of graded responses and staged indicators requires decentralized decision-making.

Data collection and analysis can be made more efficient by concentrating on the most susceptible families and individuals, known as a "sentinel" sample. The types of variable that are most often relevant include rainfall, crop conditions and prospects, livestock status, food prices, employment, and nutritional status. Measurements of nutritional status (usually meaning anthropometry) may be used as a trigger mechanism to initiate urgent relief operations if earlier interventions are not fully effective and to identify (target) areas where relief and rehabilitation measures are necessary.

Purposes and Definitions

A timely warning and intervention programme is designed to mitigate periodic household food shortages and thus prevent famines. It need not be designed to cope with or relieve famines (see ref. *1* and *2*) because it should prevent them. But surveillance will only help to prevent famines if its function is clearly related to this objective and if it is not turned into a multipurpose exercise. The limited experience to date of applying nutritional surveillance to prevent acute food shortages emphasizes this point. Nutritional surveillance for this purpose should in fact be a programme of intervention supported by information.

There is no reason why this concept should be limited to prevention of food shortages on the scale of famines. It is equally relevant to localized short-term food shortages, possibly more so, since these tend to be less known. Such events are usually seasonal and may involve a worsening of regular "hungry" seasons.

These two considerations – the need to integrate interventions and information, and the need to apply them to acute food shortages, whether or not these are regarded as famines – lead us to propose that this aspect of nutritional surveillance should be referred to as *timely warning and intervention programmes to prevent acute food shortages*. This also helps to define the relationship of nutritional surveillance to activities such as crop forecasting. We regard prevention of acute food shortages, with their consequent risk of epidemic malnutrition, as within our concern when a programme is set up to deal with this problem. One purpose of this chapter is to try to clarify concepts on the basis of recent experience, and to set out methods both of intervention and of relevant information-gathering that may be useful for wide application.

The establishment of timely warning and intervention programmes is worth while, it is suggested, when all three of the following conditions are satisfied:

– there is a risk of intermittent acute food shortages affecting certain parts of the population;

– the resources and organization are available (or potentially so) for interventions to be undertaken to prevent these shortages;

– there is a lack of adequate information to trigger these interventions.

Acute food shortages can be prevented either by decreasing the vulnerability of a susceptible population or by predicting the food consumption shortage and intervening to make up the deficit. Decreasing vulnerability to acute food shortages is clearly the long-term solution. Information collected to predict food shortages will be useful for this purpose. However, other information required to achieve this objective, and its use, is similar to that discussed in Chapter 4, and will not be repeated here. We will deal only with timely prediction or detection of food consumption shortages for intervention in the short term.

Both a predictive capability and a response mechanism are needed to prevent acute food consumption shortages. Both of these require a knowledge of the causes of decreased food consumption. Are the causes due to inadequate home food production, inadequate market availability of food at usual prices, inadequate income to purchase food, or a combination of these? Depending on the causes, interventions can include supplying agricultural inputs, price stabilization, public works programmes, and food distribution; these are discussed in detail in the next section. The most important link in the prediction-intervention chain is a mechanism that automatically triggers the initiation of the necessary intervention when the information is received.

A timely warning and intervention programme depends critically on timeliness of data collection and analysis, and on fast and efficient linkages to decision-making. Essentially it is necessary to allow sufficient time to initiate an intervention and for the intervention to take effect, in order to prevent a predicted deterioration in food consumption. A timely warning and intervention programme might be set up by modifying or adding to a system that is already operational for long-term monitoring or programme evaluation. In practice, this has not been the approach, and the programmes reviewed here have been or are being instituted specifically for the purpose of timely warning.

Timely warning and intervention programmes are useful only where there is a risk of acute food shortage and where the necessary interventions can be implemented but their implementation is liable to be hindered by a lack of information. These considerations are important in estimating the costs of collecting and analysing data quickly enough for them to be used predictively and weighing these costs against possible benefits of using the same resources for reducing the vulnerability of the area surveyed. In many cases, efforts can be concentrated in those areas that are especially vulnerable to acute food shortage. This requires that a preliminary effort be made to identify these areas.

Response and type of information collected are another important consideration. Clearly, there is little point in predicting food shortage if there are no mechanisms available with which to respond. The type of response available and the speed with which it can be implemented determine the type and periodicity of information needed. When the response includes importing food (either bought on the international market or as food aid) the required lead time may be substantially lengthened. On the other hand, in countries such as Indonesia, where food shortages are much smaller in scale and resources are available, interventions require a much shorter lead time and thus the need for advance notice is decreased. The information needed must therefore be carefully selected to fit the range of responses and re-examined as interventions change.

In principle, making a system function involves three time-periods, each of which may be open to change through improved efficiency (see Fig. 6.1):

1. The period between change in an indicator and detection of the change ((a) to (b) in Fig. 6.1); this is the lag period due to data flow and analysis.

2. The period needed to decide on, organize, and initiate an intervention ((b) to (c) in Fig. 6.1); this may be due both to bureaucratic delays and to the time required to mobilize physical resources (food, agricultural inputs, equipment for public works, etc.).

3. The period of start-up and implementation of the intervention before it has the desired stabilizing effect on food consumption.

Evidently these time-periods vary depending on the intervention, although not much seems to be known about this.

One fact should, however, be obvious. Timely warning and intervention programmes are stop-gap measures and are no substitute for other efforts to discover the fundamental causes of vulnerability. Thus the long-term solution is not to set up a timely warning and intervention programme, however effective it may be, but to abolish the need for one.

Fig. 6.1. Illustration of some concepts in timely warning and intervention

Predictive indicator

Food consumption

Result of intervention

Intervention

Level of food consumption requiring relief

Time

(a) (b) (c) (d)

Monitor effectiveness of intervention

Predictive indicator changes

Intervention initiated

Change in indicator detected

Intervention effective

Data flow and analysis

Time needed for intervention to take effect

Lead-time needed to initiate intervention

WHO 83653

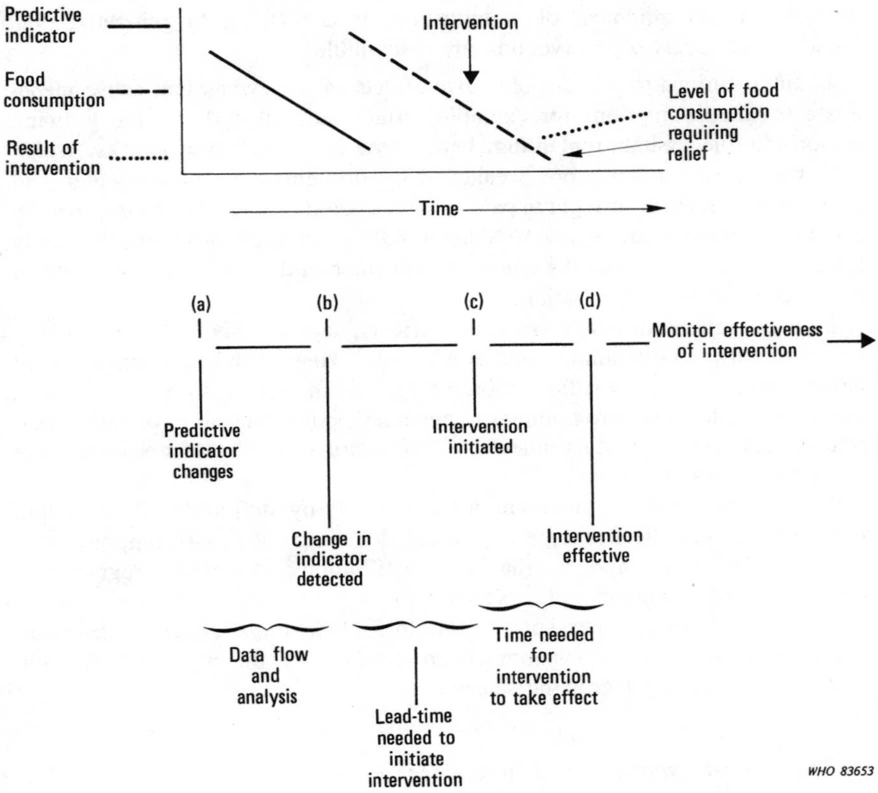

Decisions to be Taken

Decisions in a timely warning and intervention programme relate to certain predefined activities that have already been planned in case they are necessary. They thus differ from activities to be initiated on the basis of the previously described nutritional surveillance, which are generally not predefined in this way (Chapters 3–5). Another characteristic of these decisions is that they are staged according to the appropriate timing of a need for more information or for appropriate interventions.

Interventions and their timing

In theory, a whole range of interventions could be appropriate at different stages of a developing food shortage. Which interventions are made will depend largely on the causes of the shortage and on whether they are undertaken early; later interventions will tend to be more of a standard character – e.g., food distribution and treatment of malnutrition. It is difficult to generalize, but broadly four levels of intervention are discernible:

1. Interventions to prevent the basic effects of the events that cause inadequate food consumption: for example, erratic rainfall early in the growing season may necessitate replanting, hence seed is needed; pest attacks, which may particularly affect crops weakened by drought, call for pesticides and equipment; effects of drought in pastoral areas could conceivably be lessened by providing animal feed; income loss due to falling prices of cash crops (normally for exports) could be eased by government intervention to subsidize producer prices or provide compensation.

2. Interventions to attack secondary effects, such as loss of income, rising consumer prices, dwindling food stocks, etc. These would be implemented before food consumption falls substantially. Examples of such interventions might be public works programmes to generate income, subsidies of staple food prices, subsidized marketing of less-preferred staples, moving of stocks of staple foods into the area, etc.

3. The third type of intervention is needed, by definition, if preceding interventions have been unable to prevent declining food consumption. Such interventions are the more familiar food distribution and feeding programmes, rehabilitation programmes, etc. (see ref. 1).

4. A fourth set of interventions should include those aimed at relieving longer-term effects and preventing recurrences – e.g., the supply of seed and pesticides for the next growing season.

Combining interventions and indicators

The purpose and function of a timely warning and intervention programme is to combine the organization and resources needed for the various interventions with the information to run them effectively. This gives clear requirements for, and limits to, predictive information. The need is only for triggering interventions, not for prediction for its own sake. A theoretical example is given in Fig. 6.2. In this figure, a possible sequence of events is shown in which an acute food shortage is caused by drought. This is merely to exemplify what we are talking about, and does not represent real data or any particular situation. The first graph in the figure indicates a deficit and delay in rainfall. This could be presented as accumulated deficit, as shown in the second graph. (A more useful calculation in practice is to use a water balance or rainfall index, as discussed on pp. 187–189). Normally, this would be likely to lead to a decrease in food production, which can be shown as a food production rate (third graph). At the same time, food stocks will be depleted, maybe more rapidly due to droughts in previous years (fourth graph). At this stage, if the need were recognized, it

Fig. 6.2. Examples of sequence of indicators (hypothetical)

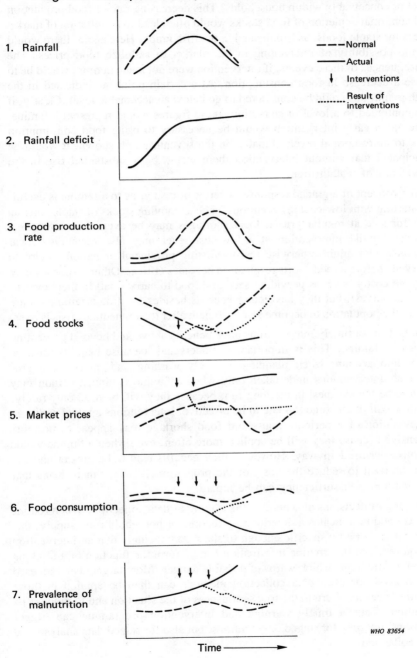

1. Rainfall

2. Rainfall deficit

3. Food production rate

4. Food stocks

5. Market prices

6. Food consumption

7. Prevalence of malnutrition

– – – Normal
—— Actual
↓ Interventions
········ Result of interventions

Time ⟶

WHO 83654

might be possible to intervene to build up food stocks again, either at the area level or conceivably within households. This decreasing rate of food production and abnormal depletion of food stocks would often lead to an inflation of market prices for staple foods, as is indicated in the fifth graph. Here again, there would be the possibility of intervening in the market to stabilize food prices. The consequences of these events, if intervention were not made in time, would be to cause a decrease in food consumption. At a certain point, as indicated in the sixth graph, this could be considered to go below an acceptable level. Clearly, if this continued to a level of starvation, these figures would represent a famine. Here again early intervention would be necessary to bring food consumption back to more normal levels. Finally, in the seventh graph shown, it would be anticipated that without intervention there would be a substantial rise in the prevalence of malnutrition.

The concept of a graded response or series of responses to a famine is useful. By starting with low-cost interventions, such as moving stocks of staples into an area for sale at regular prices, local shortages may be averted without great expense. Initial intervention at a low-cost level may also encourage local officials, who might otherwise resist enlisting provincial or national help, to intervene before a food shortage situation becomes critical. Other responses may be more costly, such as providing seed and food to carry small farmers over to the next harvest, but they have other benefits besides averting a famine – they permit the population to become self-sufficient after the immediate crisis is over.

In fact, most timely interventions have benefits above and beyond preventing a specific famine. This is important to understand, because benefits must be taken into account when planning a timely warning and intervention pro-gramme. Interventions undertaken only when a famine is almost certain may seem to be the cheapest in the long run, because they will be used only rarely, but they will often come too late to be effective. Interventions applied earlier in the evolution of a periodic household food shortage may appear to be more expensive because they will be applied more often, even when a famine would not have occurred anyway. However, their benefits tend to be greater and can often be used to reduce the costs of the programme. Thus, timely loans that permit future self-sufficiency can be repaid.

Staging of decisions also permits the staging of data collection. When routine data collection indicates a deteriorating income or household food supply, this information is rarely specific enough to show convincingly that an intervention is required. But this routine information can perform the function of a blinking yellow traffic light, which warns of possible danger. More targeted and focused data analysis or even data collection methods can then be applied in those circumstances to ascertain the true seriousness of the situation and to monitor its evolution. Thus a timely warning and intervention programme can trigger decisions, not only for staged interventions, but also for staged data analysis and data collection.

Targeting is another issue that concerns the administration of famine interventions. Some interventions, such as making available at a subsidized price low-status staple foods like cassava, or low grades of rice, will be self-targeting, because only the very poor will want to participate. When massive supplemental feeding using regular staples is necessary, other methods of targeting may need to be used. If supplemental food is distributed it is important that tribal, religious, or other group differences do not exclude recipients. In the Sahel famine, food distribution through agriculturalist village leaders often missed pastoralists who had less access to this type of aid (3).

Organization

While the individual responses of different governments to acute food shortages must necessarily be specific both to the problem and to the country's resources, there are some general conclusions that can be drawn from past experience. Since time is often critical, and since local officials have more complete information on their area of jurisdiction than would be available higher up the bureaucracy, it is probably useful both to initiate requests and to administer interventions at as low an administrative level as possible. This is the approach proposed by the Indonesian nutritional surveillance system, with its use of regency heads as initiators and administrators of local interventions. In Botswana, an attempt was made to set up district drought committees responsible to District Commissioners, to monitor "incidence of drought and drought relief" (4). Each committee formulated its own indicators with little guidance from the national level as to what sources of information were either available or potentially useful. The committees were not able to determine precisely what criteria would induce the national government to supply interventions or the funds for them, and since they had no resources of their own or access to a national coordinating body, they were not very effective. The answer to such problems seems to lie in a balance between local decision-making and accountability on the one hand, and national-level inputs of resources, guidance and coordination of sectoral data collection, and intervention assistance on the other. This may require that certain resources be kept in hand in case a deterioration in the future is indicated. The resources can be budgetary, e.g., for public works, or physical, e.g., food. The reluctance of administrators to keep resources available is understandable and a similar problem is encountered with other types of "disaster preparedness". This problem will be solved only by careful calculation of risks and trade-offs in individual cases. Such calculations should be made at an early stage of planning – because specific interventions and the required resources must be identified in advance – and only if adequate resources can be set aside or diverted can the programme be established.

The coordination of data collection, flow and analysis with data interpretation and use for deciding about the interventions is crucial to an effective timely warning and intervention programme. Many of the relevant data come from various sources, collected within different agencies. These data usually serve other purposes besides those of warning, and the programme management cannot usually exert much authority over their relevance and the quality of collection. Although the programme can arrange for more rapid data flow and analysis to the extent that this is done with programme resources, it appears that certain data *collection* must be made specifically under the authority of the programme, whether or not this is done through other agencies. However, for a timely warning and intervention programme to collect routinely all possible relevant data would not only duplicate other data-collection mechanism but would also be inefficient, because much of the information would only be needed when the decision requiring that information had to be made. Reserving such data collection for situations when there is a real need for it (i.e., when a specific intervention is under consideration) permits a staged and focused use of resources.

Data Requirements

The data requirements are determined by the need to decide whether to set predefined activities in motion.

Indicators

The methodology of nutritional surveillance *(5)* discusses "early" and "later" indicators. This breakdown could be expanded into early, concurrent, and later indicators to trigger required interventions, rather than to predict deteriorating food consumption. The terms "early", "concurrent" and "later" refer, therefore, to the time of decision, not to the food shortage or famine itself. Household food storage levels, for instance, are an early indicator when they are used to predict deteriorating nutritional status and a concurrent indicator when used to measure the severity of a food shortfall.

In Table 6.1, an example is given of the timing of interventions by early and concurrent indicators. In practice, the present use by administrators is that early indicators are taken as a warning to prepare for intervention, and this is initiated when confirmation is received from a concurrent indicator. For example (see Table 6.1), evidence that rainfall failure might cause extensive crop damage during germination might lead an administrator to take the first steps towards emergency measures to distribute seed. The actual distribution itself would often be delayed until germination failure was confirmed. Finally, it is important to know that the seed distribution worked and that the crop is progressing satisfactorily. This stresses that indicators are relevant to producing the required action.

Table 6.1. Examples of interventions linked to indicators

Examples of indicators used to initiate each intervention		Examples of interventions to be initiated
Early indicators	Concurrent indicators	
Rainfall deficit during vulnerable period in crop cycle	Failure of crop to germinate	Seed (or credit) for replanting
Failed crop or other income failure	Decreased food purchasing	Public works employment programme
Decreased food intake	Increased malnutrition	Food distribution

Sentinel samples

Very often the evaluation of developing household food shortages follows a similar pattern if recurrent food shortages are due to the same causes. For instance, if drought is the usual cause, some areas are more likely to be affected than others. Harvest deficits will affect stocks and purchasing power, and hence ability to sustain nutrition, more in some families than in others. Also, some family members are more susceptible to a deterioration in nutritional status than others. These particularly susceptible areas, families and individuals can therefore give early warning, as does a sentinel, of changes that may later affect those less susceptible. Sampling of these sentinel areas, families and individuals should lighten the burden of data collection and analysis considerably.

The concept of a sentinel sample is closely coupled to that of staging in data collection. Nationwide routine data on income-producing activities and food availability can identify areas that need more careful monitoring. Analysis of more specific routine indicators in these areas, concentrating on sentinel subareas and sentinel subgroups in these areas, can identify times when more specific data collection is required to confirm the existence of a problem or to monitor its evolution.

It is the combination of the appropriate indicator and its collection in the appropriate sentinel group at the right stage for the decision to be made that determines the usefulness of the data for a timely warning and intervention programme.

Specific types of data, their collection and presentation

Rainfall is clearly of fundamental interest when acute food shortages result from drought. Rainfall measurements are easier to interpret when information is available on historical trends and potential evapotranspiration, since this allows calculation of periods of water shortage for crops. Data for calculation of evapotranspiration rates, and thus of water balances, can be collected by agricultural or meteorological stations, and take into account temperature, relative humidity, sunshine duration, and wind speed, so as to give a more accurate picture of what damage is likely to ensue from lack of rain. Since this information is much less variable than rainfall itself, evapotranspiration data can be collected at a central station and used for interpreting rainfall data collected from surrounding areas of similar geography and cropping.

In Botswana, rainfall data are reported from schools. This may be a satisfactory low-cost way of collecting such information; measurement is not difficult with the right equipment, and using schools ensures wide coverage. Drawbacks to the system include making arrangements for collection and reporting during breaks and holidays, and the cost of diverting school resources for this purpose.

Current rainfall data are useful as an early indicator of famine when presented not only against a backdrop of previous trends, but also when analysed in conjunction with additional agricultural information, such as crops planted, planting dates, and soil types. Studies from India, for example, using yearly yield and rainfall data between 1932 and 1964, have shown that while there is no correlation between total seasonal rainfall and yields, the distribution of rainfall (calculated, for example, over 10-day periods) is critical. Again, looking at the data from a 32-year period in Senegal and using an index system that considers cropping patterns, planting dates, soil type, and rainfall distribution as well as totals, a good correlation was seen (see Fig. 6.3) *(6)*, whereas no correlation with total rainfall was found. Another problem with the use of rainfall data alone, even disaggregated by 10-day periods, is that shifts in the rainy season by as much as a month are not uncommon, e.g., in the Sahel. If planting is delayed until the rains start, and if the season extends long enough for harvest, then what would appear, by the analysis of rainfall data alone, to be a disaster, could, in the light of planting dates, prove to be no problem.

Crop conditions and prospects can thus be monitored using data on planting dates and other crop-cycle information, integrated with rainfall data. In Ethiopia, this type of information is collected by farmers' associations, and this may be a useful, low-cost system if such organizations are available. When the main risk factor is drought, it is probable that rainfall measurements combined with reporting on crop progress through different stages of growth could provide one of the basic methods for early warning. Thus crop-forecasting systems are often considered as similar to, or part of, nutritional surveillance systems. Many of the data proposed in the Joint FAO/UNICEF/WHO Expert Committee report *(5)* for providing early indicators in subsistence cropping systems (e.g., see Table 3 on page 29 of that report) are normally regarded as part of crop-forecasting systems. Their main use at present is to support national policies on agricultural imports and exports, pricing, storage, etc. They are not usually linked with interventions to prevent effects on food consumption of forecasts of crop shortfalls. They could therefore contribute to nutritional surveillance timely warning and intervention programmes but are not the same as these. Crop-fore-

Fig. 6.3. Example of use of indexing to interpret rainfall data [a,b]

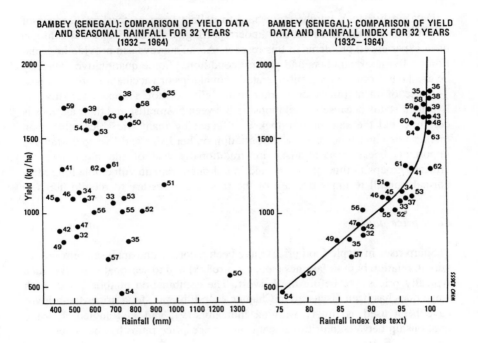

BAMBEY (SENEGAL): COMPARISON OF YIELD DATA AND SEASONAL RAINFALL FOR 32 YEARS (1932–1964)

BAMBEY (SENEGAL): COMPARISON OF YIELD DATA AND RAINFALL INDEX FOR 32 YEARS (1932–1964)

[a] Source: Frere & Popov (6, p. 22). Reproduced by permission of the Food and Agriculture Organization of the United Nations.
[b] The figures beside each point indicate the year in which the comparison was made.

casting systems have been established in many developing countries (e.g., Algeria, Argentina, Bangladesh, Ethiopia, Kenya, Nepal, Senegal, United Republic of Tanzania, and others) on either a pilot or a national basis. It is worth noting that in no case, even in developed countries, are the high-technology methods of satellite observation yet used routinely for crop forecasting, although they are used to monitor the risk of locust plagues.

In the context of predicting crop forecasts, the drought-warning system in Australia, which has been operating since 1965 to monitor rainfall deficits, is of particular interest (7). The system was computerized in 1974, and includes data from 800 selected meteorological stations that have been reporting for over 40 years. By comparing current data with historical trends the system is able to tell some twenty days before the end of the month which areas are definitely not experiencing a rainfall deficit, which areas are marginal, and which have a ' statistical probability of not reaching a specified cut-off level of rain' monthly period.

Livestock status

Data on livestock numbers are hard to collect from pastoralists because of migration, division of herds, and underreporting. Both Botswana and Ethiopia have experienced problems in this respect. Aerial surveys can provide information on livestock numbers and pasture conditions. Some quantitative data may be available from government-operated animal dips or vaccination programmes. The use of meat prices or market availability is not a good alternative to livestock status because the relationship between pastoralist and their animals is complex and the sale of livestock is affected by many variables other than market price and food scarcity. Information on herd size and livestock status is important, because pastoralists are traditionally one of the most severely affected groups in time of famine and in a drought remain vulnerable long after normal rainfall resumes because of the time lag necessary to rebuild herds.

Food price data

Sharp rises in staple food prices have been recorded and analysed retrospectively in relation both to famines (see, e.g., ref. *8*) and to seasonal scarcity, when typically prices rise before the harvest. The combination of food prices with wage rates has been discussed in Chapter 4. In Ethiopia, food prices themselves have been used as timely warning indicators (*9*), and in Bangladesh some relationship between nutritional status and wage/price ratios has been observed (see Table 6.2).

There can be problems associated with both collection of price data and their interpretation. Reported prices may depend on the person who collects the data. In many countries, staple food prices are controlled by legislation, hence reporting of actual prices may be difficult. None the less, retail price reporting is widely undertaken and is a promising source of raw data for early warning.

Interpretations of price data will vary depending on the causes of food consumption crises. If supply in the market is the constraint, price rises would be expected to reflect declining food consumption; however, if the problem is lack of income with adequate market supply – as is expected to be the case in Indonesia – the price of the primary staples might give no indication of consumption problems. In extreme cases the price could even fall. Certainly shift of consumption to secondary staples (e.g., cassava in Indonesia) might be expected, and this might be the price to monitor[1] instead of the price of the primary staple. Thus interpretation of price changes will be specific to individual situations and will require a detailed understanding of the economic behaviour involved.

---

[1] See DAPICE, D. *Analytical issues in indicator and intervention preparation of the Indonesia Nutritional Surveillance System*. Ithaca, NY, Cornell University, 1980 (Cornell Nutritional Surveillance Program) (mimeographed document).

Table 6.2. Price-wage ratios (real wages) compared with prevalence of second- and third-degree malnutrition among children under 10 years of age in A-class families in famine-prone areas of Bangladesh (June to September 1979) [a]

Location	Unit price of rice in takas (a_1)	Daily wage (without food) in takas (a_2)	Real wage[b] $= \dfrac{a_2}{a_1}$	Percentage of children with IInd- and IIIrd-degree malnutrition[b,c]
Kurigram (Rangpur)	6.75	8.00	1.19	47.62(42)
Sirajgani (Pabna)	5.87	4.50	0.77	32.0 (25)
Matlab (Comilla)	5.50	9.30	1.73	27.27(33)
Shibchar (Faridpur)	6.25	6.25	1.00	31.71(41)
Goalandaghat (Faridpur)	6.48	10.00	1.54	21.21(33)
Sandwip (Chittagong)	6.87	11.00	1.60	40.0 (50)
Rajoir (Faridpur)	6.75	8.00	1.19	32.43(37)
Chilmari (Rangpur)	7.25	5.50	0.76	56.25(48)
Sadullapur (Rangpur)	6.10	5.00	0.82	56.67(60)
Bauphal (Patuakhali)	7.37	16.00	2.17	20.45(44)

[a] Source: Ahmad, K. On nutritional surveillance. Paper delivered at the Third Asian Congress on Nutrition, 6-10 October, 1980, at Jakarta, Indonesia.
[b] Correlation coefficient $= -0.69$, $P < 0.5$, between last two columns.
[c] Figures in parentheses show the total number of children under 10 years of age in the corresponding village. (Total number in all villages: 413.)

Employment data

Employment data could be used as early indicators of impending food consumption crises; indeed, their use for this purpose is being investigated in Indonesia. A marked increase in unemployment in an area vulnerable to food consumption crises would reflect a fall in purchasing power – whether the income loss was due directly to crop failure (i.e., for the small farmer himself or for the labourer put out of work by the farmer's loss of income) or to other economic changes, such as large shifts in producer prices. Here, again, some detailed knowledge of the economics of the specific situation is required to choose indicators and interpret changes in them.

Nutritional status

There are essentially four uses for nutritional status data in a timely warning and intervention programme. First, it is likely that in many cases early preventive interventions may not be fully effective, and some monitoring of nutritional status may be needed as a back-up.

Secondly, nutritional status data can be used to trigger urgent relief operations, because by the time nutritional status is affected, a life-threatening food shortage has progressed dangerously far. Routinely collected clinical data may not be dependable for this purpose because clinics may not be serving the most vulnerable households or members of households. Surveys directed specifically at such households or individuals are more likely to pick up the changes in nutritional status, which include weight-for-height and clinical signs, and should trigger household or area food or income relief or possibly both. These household surveys need only be instituted when other surveillance data give a "yellow light" warning that an area is becoming endangered. They are therefore under the authority of the programme and can be designed and standardized both in their measurements and in their sampling of households and persons.

Thirdly, and related to the first use, nutritional status is the obvious basis for targeting relief and rehabilitation measures. In some situations, for instance, in Botswana, relief is a main purpose of the system, and thus nutritional status is the most-used indicator. In some circumstances, one way to build up a timely warning and intervention programme might even be to start from nutritional status data and ensure that relief is delivered where it is needed, developing as fast as possible to preventive intervention. Of the possible nutritional status indicators weight-for-height is probably the most useful for representing current food shortages. Weight-for-age or height-for-age are probably too dependent on past chronic food shortages – which may be common in drought-prone areas – to characterize recent malnutrition accurately. Further, reliable records of age are sometimes hard to obtain. Birth-weight data, if available, would also reflect decreased food consumption – especially in the last three months of pregnancy.

Fourthly, nutritional status data should be useful for defining areas of vulnerability. Areas with chronic malnutrition will sometimes be more vulnerable to superimposed acute food shortages; this depends on ecology, etc., and will not apply in all cases. Other indicators, therefore, will often be needed. An example of where the relationship between chronic and acute malnutrition might not hold would be in higher rainfall areas where food supply is fairly stable but infection causes poor nutritional status; in drier areas, in non-drought years, nutritional status might be good, but vulnerability would still be high. This would probably be the picture going north from sub-Sahelian areas – say with more than 1000 mm rainfall per year – to drier areas – say less than 500 mm rainfall – in West Africa.

If clinic data are used it is important to realize that along with the usual biases, pastoralists will probably be underrepresented and sample surveys may need to be undertaken in order to investigate their nutritional status. This is an example of the more general problem, that particular subgroups in the population may be affected but not well represented in the data.

Nutritional status data are most useful when presented against time-series data which show normal seasonal trends. If the data are available regularly from clinics, then some attempt should be made to use them for targeting and monitoring of interventions. Because of the relatively slow rate of change in nutritional status and the outcome nature of the variable itself, monthly reporting and analyses would probably suffice. In areas where large amounts of anthropometric data are available from clinics, sampling techniques can be used to make the statistics more manageable. An analysis of percentage of children at risk or below a certain cut-off point, together with the change in percentage for the same area from previous months or years, might be useful. However, because of sampling and coverage differences it is difficult to make statements about relative differences between regions or reporting areas. This problem is compounded in pastoral areas and by general migration due to food shortages.

Other uses of timely warning data

Data collected for timely warning and intervention may have some uses for either monitoring and evaluation or long-term planning purposes. The latter may be particularly useful in directing resources towards decreasing the vulnerability of different groups to events likely to lead to famine. Other uses of early warning data include documentation for requests for international emergency aid and for the monitoring of interventions themselves. In addition, in the aftermath of a famine, the kinds of data available through early warning systems may prove useful for targeting for rehabilitation.

REFERENCES

1. PROTEIN-CALORIE ADVISORY GROUP FOR THE UNITED NATIONS SYSTEM. *A guide to food and health relief operations for disasters*. New York, United Nations, 1977.
2. DE VILLE DE GOYET, C. ET AL. *The management of nutritional emergencies in large populations*. Geneva, World Health Organization, 1978.
3. SHEETS, H. & MORRIS, R. *Disaster in the desert – failure of international relief in the West African drought*. Washington, DC, The Carnegie Endowment for International Peace, 1974 (Humanitarian Policy Studies, Special Report).
4. WILY, E. An aspect of warning systems for drought: information collecting in the districts. In: Hinchley, M. T., ed. *Symposium on drought in Botswana*. Hanover, NH, The Botswana Society (distributed by the University Press of New England), 1979, pp. 210-218.

5. WHO Technical Report Series, No. 593, 1976 *(Methodology of nutritional surveillance. Report of a Joint FAO/UNICEF/WHO Expert Committee).*

6. FRERE, M. & POPOV, G. F. *Agrometeorological crop monitoring and forecasting.* Rome, Food and Agriculture Organization of the United Nations, 1979 (FAO Plant Production and Protection Paper, No. 17).

7. LEE, D. M. Australian drought watch system. In: Hinchley, M. T., ed. *Symposium on drought in Botswana.* Hanover, NH, The Botswana Society (distributed by the University Press of New England), 1979, pp. 173-187.

8. SEAMAN, J. & HOLT, J. Markets and famines in the third world. *Disasters*, **4**: 283-297 (1980).

9. ETHIOPIA. *Food supply system report, vol. 2, No. 3, June-August 1978.* Addis Ababa, Relief and Rehabilitation Commission, 1978.